YOGA FOR HEALTH AND BEAUTY

Joan Gould has been interested in yoga ever since she was a small girl and has studied and practised it most of her life. She realized the full extent of the value of yoga in 1962 when her husband was stricken with a near-fatal heart attack in a remote part of the north of Italy far from all contacts and friends. Mrs Gould joined him for three months, during which time she taught yoga and also visited the Yesudian School of Yoga in Switzerland. It became clear to her that the mental benefits of yoga are considerable. On her return home she continued to teach it and has done so ever since. Now widowed, she lives in the country with her four children. Of her present life, she says, 'I enjoy all the beauties of nature, walking barefoot on the grass, cycling, tennis, bridge, cooking, sewing, painting and collecting antiques. I do not like artificiality, crowds, city life, late nights and post offices.'

YOGA
for Health and Beauty

JOAN GOULD

PAN BOOKS LTD
LONDON AND SYDNEY

First published 1969 by Thorsons Publishers Ltd
This edition published 1974 by Pan Books Ltd,
Cavaye Place, London SW10 9PG

ISBN 0 330 24015 3

Printed in Great Britain by
Fletcher & Son Ltd, Norwich

Acknowledgements

In accordance with the aims of this book, it was felt that all the illustrations should be as natural as possible, thus in compliance with my request various women students graciously consented to demonstrate the postures and the photographs were taken out-of-doors in my garden. I think they have demonstrated very ably that the postures are within reach of all.

I wish to express my sincere thanks to them for their co-operation, and also to my son Charles who took most of the photographs.

JOAN GOULD

Contents

Introduction

MUCH has been written in the past about Yoga in all its branches—so much so that most people are now familiar with the subject and know that the form of physical Yoga which we are going to discuss is properly known as HATHA YOGA. For the sake of convenience I am going to drop the "HATHA" from the name and will refer to Hatha Yoga as YOGA from now onwards.

Yoga has interested me for many years, and knowing what a wonderful elixir it is, I have been delighted to instruct other women in the art so that they too may enjoy all the benefits which the breathing, exercises and relaxation bring. The Yoga that I have taught has been simple and straightforward and eminently suited to women of today, enabling them to make it part of their everyday lives. Many of my pupils have said that it would be of great value to have a comprehensible handbook, fully illustrated, covering the instructions for breathing, for the exercises, for the system of breath control combined with the exercises and for complete relaxation. You will observe that there is no reference at all to the spiritual branch of Yoga in this book. This is quite deliberate and the omission has been made for two reasons. Firstly, I find there are very few women who wish to delve into this aspect of Yoga, most of them being interested in the health angle, and secondly, I feel instructions of this nature should come from dedicated Gurus (teachers) who live in ashrams in India and who devote their entire lives to the complete study of Yoga in its spiritual form. Should your interest in Yoga take you as far as this, you will have no difficulty in finding suitable guidance in the many books which have been written covering this subject.

My belief is that we should take the best from the age-old Yoga system of physical culture, and sift out that which is most suitable for women to help maintain and improve health, beauty and temperament, so that with this object in view this book has been compiled to enable all women everywhere, no matter what their occupation or creed, to enrich their lives by the practice of Yoga.

The book has been set out in two parts in an endeavour to make the instructions as clear as possible. Part One deals with the specialised system of health breathing and exercises (which are, in turn, combined with breath control), whilst Part Two takes care of such matters as relaxation, diet, etc. All of the actual instructions are accompanied by natural photographs, making it a simple matter to understand fully how to practise at home without difficulty. Further, the benefits resulting from the practice of each exercise have been clearly set out, thus it will be easy for the student to choose those exercises most suitable for her. You will observe that the exercises given are not those associated with contortionists, but they have been carefully selected from the many known Yoga exercises so that they are suitable for you and for me—everyday women living everyday lives. I would stress that the exercises must be done without strain of any kind, and that there is no need to do each and every exercise in the book. Read through the entire book first and then go back and select those exercises which you feel are suitable for you. Begin with the very simple exercises and gradually progress to those which are a little more demanding. If there is any difficulty in attaining the complete pose, do what you are able to manage comfortably and then strive to improve your ability as the months go by.

To those women who already practise Yoga, I would say that I hope this guide will fill the need for a ready reference, whilst to those who are beginners, I hope that Yoga will become part of your natural and everyday life, and that it will bring you freedom from tension, much joy and improved health.

I dedicate this book to our very courageous and health-conscious women of today!

JOAN GOULD
February, 1969

P.S. Although the book has been designed and illustrated specially for women, if you can persuade your husband to join you in your search for health and happiness there is no reason why he should not use the book as a guide, as almost all of the exercises are equally suitable for men!

PART ONE

1

Yoga !—your key to the joy of living

HAVE you ever looked at the faces of the shoppers at the next counter, your fellow travellers in the tube or in the bus queue, or behind the wheel in the early morning traffic rush? They all have the same expression—the tenseness, the frown, the "I've-got-so-much-to-do, I'm-late-already" look. Life today, especially in the towns and cities, makes the life our grandmothers lived look like a leisurely day-dream. Today, when we can travel thousands of miles in hours; when records are broken daily; when bigger and better results are expected from everyone and everything there is one driving force behind all things—speed. Fast cars and fast planes and big business all add up to ulcers, nervous tensions and insomnia. Men are not the only victims, women too have their own "rat race"—running homes, shopping, looking after the family, entertaining, gardening, doing "good works", and in general, being chauffeur, housekeeper and jack-of-all trades.

What can we do about it all? The answer is Yoga. Yoga helps us to cope with these ever-increasing demands upon health and stamina. The Yoga we are going to talk about is HATHA YOGA, which is the oldest system of physical culture in the world, but we are going to make it suitable to moderns. This is the system which has helped thousands of people to enjoy life through mental and physical well-being, despite all modern stresses and strains. Why? What does Yoga really do and how does it help? Yoga not only exercises all parts of the body, keeping muscles and nerves toned and soothed, but the specialised system of breathing relaxes the mind and the body, stimulates the circulation and brings the richly oxygenated blood to all tissues, renewing them and prolonging their youthfulness. Yoga also activates and feeds all the

3

ductless or endocrine glands, and soon the whole body responds and begins to function smoothly like a luxury machine. All this results in that wonderful acquisition, peace of mind, and as you feel more at peace within yourself, so your contacts and relationships with others will improve and you will find that the world is really quite a nice place after all. Instead of merely existing from day to day you will feel that it is good to be alive. Every day will bring greater and renewed interest and joy through glowing health and vitality.

How can you enjoy life if you perpetually feel run down, nervous and unable to cope with the demands which the modern world makes? Resolve to commence and continue to practise Yoga and this is what will happen:

You will radiate good health,

Your eyes will sparkle,

Your complexion will glow,

Your step will regain its youthful spring,

Your arteries will become elasticised and healthy,

Your system will be regulated and constipation will disappear,

Your figure will improve, and your body will become supple,

You will be able to relax.

All of these things will be yours, and they can be yours with a minimum of effort and a great deal of pleasure.

What usually happens in cases of self-neglect as we grow older? Our bodies begin to stiffen, we have digestive troubles, our complexions fade, we lose the dewy fresh look of youth, waistlines sag and our activities slow down—BUT—all this is not necessary and you should not accept reduced activity and various aches and pains as part of the process of maturity. Yoga will open the door to the secret of eternal youth—it will reverse the ageing forces of nature if you will make it part of your life. Instead of trying to patch up the ravages of shallow breathing, an over-rich diet and little or no exercise by resorting to more and more cosmetics to try and restore the bloom to your cheeks, pills to rejuvenate and slim the figure, more pills to induce tranquillity and sleep, and then more pills to alert the body again, invest a little time in working on the forces within the body through the Yoga regime, follow a wholesome diet and witness the miraculous results!

Unfortunately, many women have been discouraged from taking up Yoga because they have gained the impression through many books and through advanced demonstrations that in order to do Yoga they have to be contortionists. You do not have to tie yourself into complicated knots in order to enjoy the manifold benefits of Yoga because there are a large variety of simple postures which will bring maximum benefits, and the average woman will be able to practise these postures with ease. Then, to correct another false impression, because you are doing Yoga you do not have to withdraw from your families and friends in order to live the life of a crank or a recluse, nor will you have to devote hours of your precious time standing on your head or in doing the recommended exercises. It is not necessary to stand on your head and, in fact, I do not recommend this posture to my mature students, whilst the exercises need take up no more of your time than that which you would spend drinking a second cup of tea at the breakfast table whilst reading the paper, or gossiping with a chatty friend on the telephone.

If you wish to become an expert pianist, or crack tennis player, or golfer, you will naturally set aside time to practise. You must do the same with Yoga—practice will make perfect. You will get out of Yoga what you put into it and if you devote one hour per week to a serious session of exercises and then set aside fifteen minutes each day in an effort to perfect those postures which you particularly desire to develop, this will be sufficient to keep you feeling on top of the world. Most women are usually up and about for at least fifteen hours per day or one hundred and five hours per week, so this means that for as little as two-and-a-half hours per week you will be exchanging below-par health for every woman's birthright—RADIANT HEALTH!

2

The practice of Yoga

THERE has always been a certain air of mystery connected with Yoga, and in fact in the East there are a number of postures devoted to awakening occult and spiritual powers. However, housewives and mothers, with few exceptions, are not interested in this aspect of Yoga and fortunately this aura of mystery is gradually being dispelled as Westerners learn to distinguish from the mists the sound rules for health. Most women want to concentrate on the physical and mental benefits which result from the practice of the postures and the breathing and this is what I want to try and help them to do by setting out in this book as clearly as possible the system to follow.

There are all sorts of questions which crop up when a beginner contemplates donning tights and starting the exercises, so here are those which occur most frequently.

Am I not too old and stiff to start Yoga?

The reply is that the only time it is too late to start Yoga is when you are dead! Yoga can be started at any age, and if the exercises are carried out sensibly they can only do good. The one point to remember when you first commence Yoga is not to strain.

I thought Yoga was a religion?

Yoga is not, and it can be followed by anyone of any religion. You do not need to be a Hindu in order to enjoy the benefits of Yoga! At this stage it would be as well to point out that one who practises the cult of Yoga is a Yogi. Do not make the mistake of saying that you are practising Yogi, you are practising YOGA.

Are the exercises any different to the ones I did at gym?
Yoga differs from other forms of physical culture in that the exercises are not rapid and violent, but they are done slowly and deliberately, with concentration and combined with Yogic breathing. Certain of the postures are maintained when the final attitude has been obtained, whilst other postures are repeated progressively. The objective in doing the exercises slowly is to stretch the muscles involved and to flush them with the newly oxygenated blood which has resulted through the breathing, whilst when the muscles are relaxed upon the release of the posture the stale blood is forced out and carried away by the stimulated circulation. The postures are combined with the Yogic breathing so that as the circulation is stimulated the system becomes revitalised and wastes are whipped away and disposed of efficiently through the lungs, skin, kidneys and bowels.

The postures and breathing must be done with concentration and sincerity and a belief that they can and will do for you all that they are capable of doing. For that reason do not treat Yoga as a party cabaret turn and do not become an exhibitionist.

Do not be afraid that Yoga will make your figure unattractive by building up muscles like those of the proverbial strong man—they will bring grace and line to the body.

There are postures to strengthen and revitalise each part of the body and you will notice as you do the exercises that great attention is paid to the spine, the brain, the legs, the nerves and the internal organs. When you have completed a period of exercise you will feel restored, not exhausted, because Yoga aims at conserving and building up your energies. In this direction bear in mind that when you begin practising Yoga at home, do not overdo any of the exercises, but begin gradually and slowly build up the time you wish to maintain a posture or the number of times you wish to repeat an exercise. This is most important, as it is as bad to strain yourself and your capabilities as it is to do no exercises at all.

Will I lose weight?
This is the evergreen question dear to all feminine hearts! Answer: weight will be adjusted according to your frame and the

needs of your body. There are many exercises which stimulate the thyroid and the rate of metabolism, so that if you are overweight you will lose. On the other hand, as the body and mind learns to relax, those who are underweight will regain more normal outlines. Furthermore, as you lose weight your muscles will be toned and will not become flabby as they so often do when violent reducing diets are embarked upon.

What do I need to start Yoga?

You can begin to practise Yoga at any time without going to any expense. You will require very little clothing and the minimum of space. What you will need in plenty is fresh air and seclusion. Your clothing requirements will depend on where you are going to do the exercises. If you are going to use the privacy of your own bedroom, your wardrobe will supply a simple blouse with short sleeves and a pair of close fitting panties, but if you decide that you would prefer to do the exercises out-of-doors, then you should wear a blouse or leotard and a pair of comfortable tights. Make quite certain that you do not wear any tight underwear, and ensure as far as practicable that you will not be interrupted once you have commenced your exercises.

If you are going to do the exercises indoors, you must use a room which is well ventilated. Naturally, it is not a good idea to use one which smells of stale cigarette smoke. The ideal arrangement is to have a secluded corner out-of-doors, preferably in a garden, and the next best is to have a small room or corner of a room entirely devoted to your own use for Yoga. The actual floor space that you will need is your own length whilst lying down plus a few spare inches, and then sufficient clear width so that you can stretch both your arms out whilst lying flat on the floor. Place a suitable rug or mat down on the floor, cover that with a clean sheet or blanket, and you are ready to begin.

There are times when you should not exercise, so do not undertake the exercises immediately after a meal if you intend to do a series of exercises or some of the more strenuous ones. You must wait for one-and-a-half hours to elapse after a light meal, or two-and-a-half hours after a heavy meal. If, however, you merely wish to relieve some physical strain or tension by doing one or two of the simple exercises, there is no need to worry about these time limits. When you are menstruating you should concentrate only on the breathing and the simple head, shoulder, neck and leg exercises for the first couple of days, thereafter you may do the more difficult ones.

Yoga Breathing is an essential part of the Yoga system of exercises as all of the postures are based upon correct breathing. It will therefore be necessary for you to make yourself familiar with the breathing before you commence to learn the postures. Here, then, is how you set about it. Remember that the same time limits that apply to your exercises must elapse between meals and your breathing practices if you intend to spend some time on the breathing exercises, but you may, of course, do the deep breathing, the Tranquillising Breath and the Alternate Nostril Breathing at any time to suit your convenience.

3

The Breathing Practices

BREATH is elixir to the brain and soul and food to the body. Everything depends upon breath! It is the one thing our bodies must have constantly. Frequently through following the correct breathing practices only, great improvement has been made in health.

Take a deep breath of God's fresh air, and another, and another! It is better than champagne! Feel the resultant glow of health spread through the body. Deep and full breathing is the first step to perfect health.

Shallow breathing is the cause of a great many ills. Without a proper supply of fresh air and oxygen your bodies will be slow and sluggish. Wastes will clog the system, you will feel off-colour, your complexions will be sallow and you will feel perpetually tired. The brain, which requires far more oxygen than the body to function efficiently, will be lethargic and dull.

Although breathing is the most natural thing in the world, people seem to lose the art of correct breathing as they grow older. Ask an average adult to take in a deep breath and see how he or she responds. Usually there will be a sharp intake of air through resultantly pinched nostrils and a rapid exhalation through the mouth. This, of course, is quite wrong. The breath should be taken in slowly and deeply through the nose and exhaled slowly through the nose also. Why? Because the nose moistens, warms, and cleans the breath before it reaches the lungs, whilst the exhalation must be under control, full and complete.

It is vital for health reasons to breathe correctly. All the functions of our bodies are dependent upon a proper supply of oxygen. Our digestive processes, the maintenance and rebuilding of tissues, the production of energy and the disposal of wastes all require richly oxygenated blood, and this comes back to proper breathing and a strong and healthy heart and bloodstream. The heart and its vast system of arteries, veins and capillaries must perform tremendously important duties. The freshly oxygenated blood must be collected from the lungs and despatched to reach and feed the brain, nerves, glands and every cell of the body. Then, when the blood is laden with waste matters it has to be pumped back again on its return journey to the lungs.

Think how an increased supply of oxygen through correct breathing can help to improve our brains and bodies. With the magic panacea so freely available to all, why is it that people will not expand their lungs and take all that nature has to offer? The average person fails miserably in using anything like the possible air capacity of the lungs. Did you know that when inhaling a normal breath most people only use about one-quarter of their possible lung capacity? Double the intake and you will already feel better. Treble it and the improvement will be even more remarkable, and even then you will still have untold wealth in health to draw upon!

Not only is it necessary to fill the lungs properly, but it is equally important to empty them thoroughly if our systems are to function efficiently. If wastes are left in the lungs, you cannot fill them with good clean air. Accordingly, when you learn the deep breathing you must pay as much attention to the instructions for emptying as to those for filling the lungs.

The breathing exercises must form part of your daily Yoga practice and are usually done before the exercises. As it is easier to learn how to breathe properly whilst lying down, the instructions which follow for the deep Yogic Breath will be carried out by you whilst lying down on the practice mat, and if necessary, the breathing can also be done whilst lying in bed. Later on you will do the breathing whilst sitting down on the practice mat which is the traditional way to carry out the breathing practices.

The eyes are kept closed throughout the breathing. In this way the mind is stilled and you are able to concentrate more easily upon the breath and the "Prana" which is being drawn into the system. There is in the air that we breathe a subtle life-force or energy which is known to Yogis as "Prana". To this Prana, which is associated with a deep pink colour, is attributed many lifegiving and magical qualities, and whilst practising deep breathing you can direct the Prana to any part of the body to advantage. If there is some part of the body which you desire to improve, or some pain which you wish to alleviate, breathe in deeply and then as you breathe out consciously direct the Prana to that part of the body, concentrating all your thoughts upon it. Prana can also be stored in the Solar Plexus as energy, and once again it is done by breathing in deeply and then directing the Prana to the Solar Plexus as you breathe out. The Solar Plexus, as you probably know, is the seat of our nervous energies.

Side benefits to full deep breathing—your metabolism will be speeded up and excess weight will melt away; your sense of smell will improve.

Smoking

It would be as well to mention right here and now that smoking never improved anyone's health. If you smoke, make up your mind from this moment to STOP. Apart from being a dirty and smelly habit and most unfeminine, it clogs up the lungs, puts a strain on the heart, ruins the complexion, spoils the palate and dulls the sense of smell.

In any event, once you have begun to breathe properly I doubt whether you will want to destroy all your good work by filling your lungs with smoke.

The Deep Yogic Breath

The instructions that follow are the first to be given towards the actual learning of Yoga. The deep Yogic Breath is one of the fundamentals, so pay great attention to all the detail. It is used throughout the exercises and in between the exercises as a relaxing breath, therefore you must practise and perfect it. Make sure that you do not wear any tight clothing whilst doing the breathing, otherwise your breath will be restricted. Throughout the book I shall state the benefits to be derived from each breathing exercise or posture and this may in some instances cause repetition but will save constant cross references.

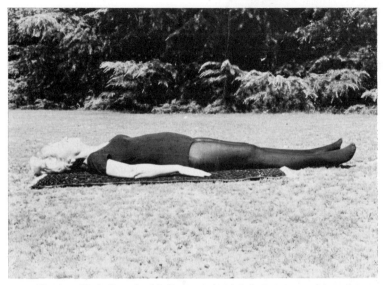

The deep Yogic Breath—(*a*) Commencing inhalation—*note abdomen.*

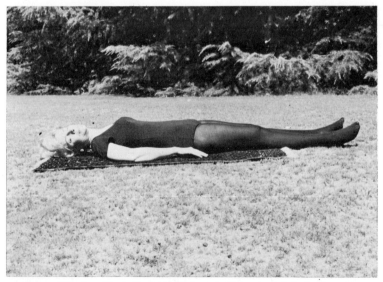

The deep Yogic Breath—(*b*) At completion on inhalation.

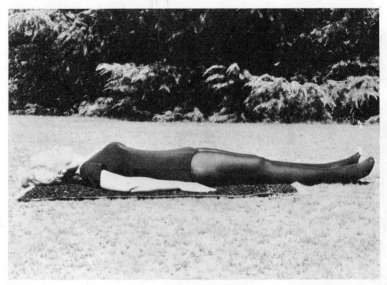

The deep Yogic Breath—(c) Completion of exhalation—*drawing abdomen in.*

Benefits

This system of breathing will improve your digestion and your circulation, and will rest your heart. Your brain, nervous system, glands and organs, in fact the whole body, will receive the tonic of a supply of newly enriched blood. At the same time your internal organs will receive the benefit of a gentle massage and you will feel relaxed and calm.

How do you breathe?

Put on your Yoga "uniform", make yourself comfortable and do not become chilled. Just before we proceed to learn the deep Yogic Breath, let us see how you breathe, so that when you have learned to breathe properly you will be able to appreciate the enormous differences between your former method and your new dynamic breath.

Do you breathe with the entire lung, making use of the upper, middle and lower sections of the lungs, or do you breathe only with the upper, or only with the middle, or only with the bottom sections? Very few adults breathe correctly. This is probably due to the fact that when we grow up and assume fashionable clothes and a "fashionable" shape, we hold ourselves incorrectly and our lungs suffer.

Lie down flat upon the back on a rug on the floor and let yourself go. Put your hands across your abdomen and begin to breathe in deeply, taking in what you normally feel is a good deep breath. Note how you are breathing and where the breath is going, and when you breathe out make sure to note the position of the abdomen. Is it pushed outwards? Then it is incorrect! Have you completed the breath? Very well, now we will compare your deep breathing with the deep Yogic Breathing. Check your position again. Be as relaxed as possible with the legs together and the feet falling outwards. Keep the hands across the abdomen, as this will help you to understand what you are doing and you will quickly notice the difference between your normal breathing and the Yoga breathing as you feel the abdomen RISING and FALL-ING as you take in and expel the breath.

In deep Yogic Breathing, ALL the lung is used—that is dynamic difference number one. The lower, middle and upper sections of the lungs are completely filled, the breath is held in for a second, then it is expelled by completely emptying the entire lung, the breath is held out for a second, and the breathing cycle is repeated again. When commencing the inhalation you will RAISE, (yes, raise), the abdomen, and when exhaling you will pull the abdomen IN, (yes, in), towards the backbone—this is dynamic difference number two. No doubt you have been breath-ing in quite the opposite way, pulling in the tummy when breathing in, and pushing it out when breathing out. Why is the correct method so different to what you have been doing in the past? Here is the explanation. Your breathing has been shallow because at the commencement of the inhalation you must raise the abdomen slightly so that the diaphragm descends and frees the lower portion of the lungs so that you are enabled to fill this area easily before taking the breath right up to the top of the lungs, whilst when you are emptying the lungs when you pull the abdomen in towards the backbone this forces the diaphragm up and so enables you to squeeze out all the stale air from the lungs.

Begin!

Empty the lungs by breathing out through the nose. (This must always be done before you start your breathing exercises.) Commence to fill the lungs, breathing in through the nose and raising the abdomen and slowly beginning to fill the lower lung. Continue to take in the breath slowly and steadily and when you have filled the lower lung continue breathing in steadily and fill the middle lung and finally the upper lung, right up to and underneath the collar bones. Whilst taking the breath in and up, the abdomen will slowly drop and assume its normal position. At the top of the inhalation after you have filled the lungs to their capacity, pause for a count of one pulse beat, and then start to exhale through the nose, emptying the upper, middle and lower lungs in the same slow continuous manner, but this time remember to pull the abdomen in well towards the backbone as you finish, thus squeezing out all the stale air.

You have taken your first DEEP YOGIC BREATH. Mark the moment well, as it is an important one in your life. Did you notice any difference between that breath and your usual shallow breathing? Almost everyone does and they are amazed at the difference in the capacity of their lungs, and the fact that they feel more alive and yet more relaxed.

Try the breath again. Make the breathing as full and as deep as possible, and this time endeavour to inhale to a slow count of SEVEN, hold the breath at the top of the inhalation for ONE pulse beat, then exhale for a slow count of SEVEN, hold the breath out for ONE pulse beat, and then continue to breathe in and out in this slow rhythmical way for up to seven full breaths. Do you not feel better already? Once you have learned to breathe properly lying down, you may begin to do the breathing whilst sitting upon the practice mat. If you are supple you will use the Lotus Seat, but at the beginning you will find that sitting in the cross-legged position is the most comfortable way. As you progress you will sit in the Half-Lotus, and then finally in the Lotus Seat. These positions are described fully in the section dealing with the Yoga Postures.

The main points to bear in mind when practising the breathing in the seated positions are:

1. Have the buttocks firmly upon the floor,
2. Keep the spine erect in a straight line with the nape of the neck,
3. Have the shoulders drawn back and slightly down,
4. Be relaxed.

If it is impossible for you to sit upon the floor, then you may sit in a straight-backed chair, placing the feet together and flat upon the floor, and once again keeping the spine erect.

The same form of breathing as has been described above should be used throughout your ordinary daily activities. Naturally the

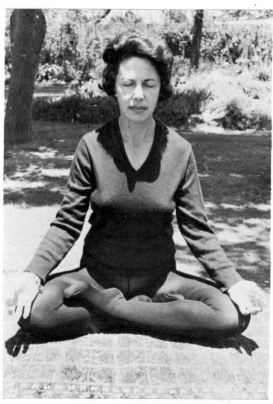

The deep Yogic Breath—sitting.

breath will not be so exaggerated, but the movements should be the same, effortless and without the pause. If you watch a small child or baby whilst it is asleep, you will see the little abdomen rising and falling in exactly the same way. This is the natural and correct way in which to breathe. The Yogis believe that in our life span we are allocated a certain number of breaths, so breathe more deeply and slowly and prolong that span.

If you wish to relax tensions during the day, make it a habit to breathe deeply whenever you have the chance. This can be done whilst you are waiting at the robot for the lights to change; whilst you are waiting for that important interview, or for your appointment at the doctor's or dentist's rooms; or when you have allowed yourself to become angry or irritated! Better still, do it before you allow yourself to become angry or irritated. The deep Yogic Breath is also used prior to Deep Relaxation, and you will find full instructions for this method of Relaxation under *The Art of Relaxation*.

The deep Yogic Breath—sitting

Early morning is the best time of all to practise your breathing, and of course the best place is out-of-doors in the fresh air. However, if it is not possible to set aside time in the early morning then do the breathing at some other time more suitable to your arrangements, and if you prefer it you may do the breathing indoors, only make certain that there is a plentiful supply of fresh air coming into the room.

Method
Sit cross-legged upon the mat. (Later you will sit in the Lotus or Half-Lotus Position.) Rest your hands upon your knees, palms up, and place the tips of the thumb and forefinger of each hand together, almost as though you were holding a flower in each hand. Ensure that your back is straight and that the nape of your neck is in line with your back. Close your eyes and then you are ready to commence your deep breathing.

Fill the lungs in the same way as you did when learning to breathe in the lying down position, that is, you raise the abdomen and fill the lower, middle and upper lungs, and then exhale whilst drawing the abdomen in towards the spine in order to empty the lungs properly. You will find it a little more difficult to carry out the deep Yogic Breath whilst sitting, but do try to make the breathing as deep and rhythmic as possible. Concentrate on drawing in the Prana for a slow count of seven, hold the breath in for one pulse beat, then exhale for a slow count of seven, hold the breath out for one pulse beat, breathe in again for seven and continue to breathe as described for the duration of the exercise. Endeavour to establish a lovely slow rhythm, breathe in and breathe out and feel the resultant peace and feeling of oneness with God's beautiful creations. Do not do too many breaths at the beginning of your practice, but increase the number gradually.

Remarks
As soon as you have completely mastered this Breath and can do it with ease, you may do an additional exercise where you extend your count to an inhalation of 7, pause 1, and exhale to a count of 14. In other words, DOUBLE THE PERIOD OF THE EXHALATION, so that the rhythm will be 7:1:14.

There are many other breathing or "Pranayama" exercises, but those which follow are among the most useful and beneficial to those of us living in the West and leading busy lives. Unless otherwise stated the exercises are done sitting upon the practice mat on the floor.

Alternate Nostril Breathing, or the nasal cleansing breath

Benefits
This breath clears the nasal passages and soothes the nerves, hence it is a good breathing exercise to do at the start of the breathing exercises. All of us have a negative and a positive current running through our bodies. These currents are constantly being balanced by the body and the Alternative Nostril Breathing assists the body in that work. You may not realise it, but we do not breathe through both nostrils at the same time. Approximately every 1 hour and forty minutes in a healthy person the breath changes, and where previously the breath was being inhaled through the right nostril, it will change and the breath will then be taken in through the left nostril. The positive breath which is

related to the right nostril is known as the "Sun" breath or the "Pingala", and the negative breath which is associated with the left nostril is known as the "Moon" breath or the "Ida". The Sun breath is warming and the Moon breath is cooling.

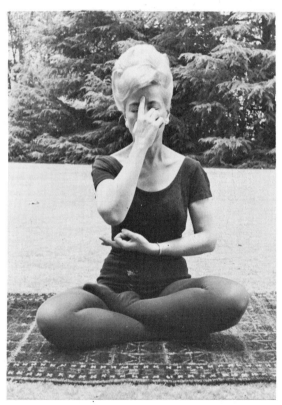

Alternate nostril breathing or the nasal cleansing breath.

Method

1. Close the circuit of the left hand by placing the tips of the thumb and forefinger together and then place the hand across the diaphragm. Ensure that the spine is held upright. Close the eyes.

2. Place the right thumb against the right nostril and close the

nostril, then inhale slowly through the left nostril for as long as you can with comfort.

3. Close both nostrils by keeping the thumb on the right nostril and closing the left nostril with the ring and little fingers of the same hand.

4. Lift the thumb and exhale slowly through the right nostril.

5. Inhale slowly through the right nostril.

6. Close both nostrils (thumb on the right nostril, and ring and little fingers on the left nostril).

7. Lift the ring and little fingers and exhale slowly through the left nostril.

This completes one round.

Remarks

You must start the inhalation with the left nostril and finish the round by exhaling through the left nostril. The breath can be done at any time of the day, and you may repeat it up to seven rounds. The breathing must be continuous, when you have completed one round begin the next round by inhaling once again through the left nostril.

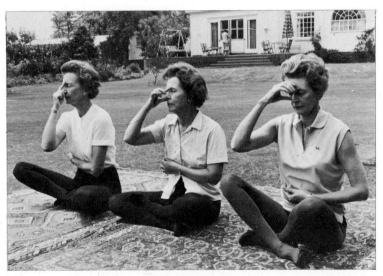

Tranquillising Breath.

Tranquillising Breath

Benefits

This breathing exercise does exactly what it says—it acts as a tranquilliser. It will also help to relieve a headache and done before retiring to bed it will help insomnia sufferers.

Method

The technique for the Tranquillising Breath is the same as that for the Alternate Nostril Breathing, differing only in the period of inhalation, retention and exhalation. Once again the breath is inhaled through the left nostril and exhaled through the right nostril, then inhaled through the right nostril and exhaled through the left nostril. The difference lies in the fact that when you inhale the breath through the left nostril take it in slowly for a count of eight, then hold the breath whilst the thumb and ring and little fingers hold the nostrils closed for a count of eight, and then exhale through the right nostril for a count of eight. Inhale once more through the right nostril for eight, hold for eight, and exhale through the left nostril for eight. This completes one round.

Remarks

The breathing must be continuous, and the next round must follow the prior round immediately. Keep the eyes closed and endeavour to establish a steady rhythm. You can practise the breath at any time during the day, and may repeat it for up to seven rounds. This breath is particularly helpful if practised when you are feeling tense or nervous, as it has a wonderful calming effect.

Breath Retention

Benefits

This breath increases the oxygenation of the blood, and calms the nervous system, whilst strengthening the lungs and the respiratory muscles.

Method

Inhale the breath for a slow count of seven through both nostrils, then hold it for as long as is comfortable concentrating on the heart and counting the beats, and then exhale again through both

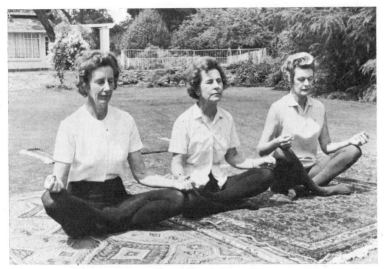

Breath Retention.

nostrils for a slow count of seven. Repeat the breath three times taking an "easy" or relaxing breath in between.

Remarks

At the beginning of your practice, you will probably only manage to hold the breath for a count of six or eight, but as your breathing becomes more efficient and your lungs strengthened, you will be able to increase the count, but do not go beyond a count of thirty-two. Before beginning the breath, ensure that you empty the lungs completely by breathing out. You may increase the number of times that the breath is repeated by one round per week, up to ten rounds. As in all the other breathing exercises, keep the eyes closed and concentrate on taking in the "Prana" and on establishing a steady rhythm.

Stimulated Breathing

Benefits

This breath brings the oxygen to all of the air cells of the lungs, consequently it improves the quality of the blood and must therefore improve all the functions of the body and appearance.

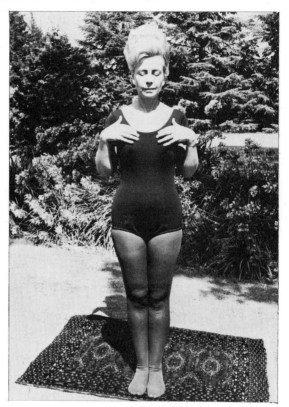

Stimulated Breathing.

Method

Stand erect with the feet together, then inhale a deep Yogic breath and whilst breathing in gently tap the chest with the tips of the fingers, running them over the complete area of the chest. After the lungs have been filled, retain the breath and whilst retaining, pat the chest with the palms of the hands, then slowly exhale through the nose. Before repeating the Stimulated Breathing, rest by taking an easy breath. You may repeat the Stimulated Breathing three times.

Remarks

Do not worry if you become a little dizzy whilst doing this breath.

If you do become dizzy, stop at once and rest a while by doing some easy breathing.

All of the breathing exercises are invaluable to smokers, and this one is particularly helpful to them.

The Breath for strengthening the nerves

Benefits
The purpose of this breath is to stimulate the nervous centres of the body and strengthen the nervous system.

Method
This breath is done in a standing position. Stand with the feet

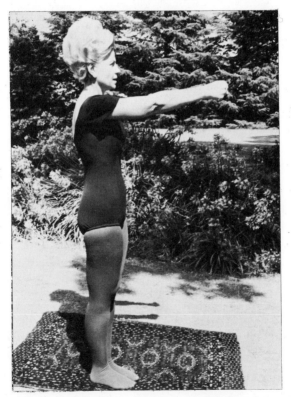

Breath for strengthening the nerves. (a) Clenching fists.

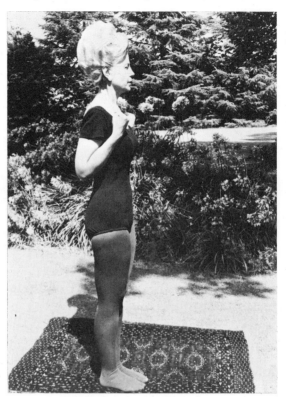

Breath for strengthening the nerves. (b) Drawing back to shoulders.

together, hands at the sides. Commence to inhale and as you do so raise the hands palms upwards in front of the body until they are level with the shoulders. Hold the breath, then clench the fists and draw them back rapidly to the shoulders; then extend the arms again and as you do so force them forward as though against great pressure; draw them back to the shoulders again and then repeat the forward movement again; repeat the drawing back and forward movements once more, then breathe out rapidly through the mouth and at the same time bend the body forward and let the hands hang down loosely. Breathe in deeply and return to starting position.

This exercise may be repeated three times.

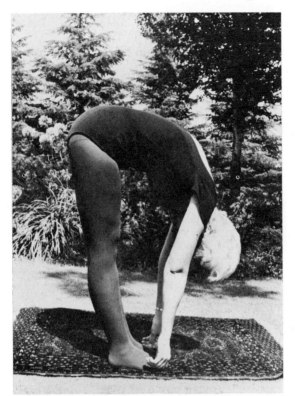

Breath for strengthening the nerves. (*c*) Breathing out.

Cleansing Breath

Benefits

This breath cleanses the lungs of any stale air and oxygenates the blood. It is particularly helpful to do this breath if you have had to spend any time in a stuffy or smoke filled room. The breath also increases the alertness of the mind.

Method

This breath is done whilst standing. Stand erect with the feet together and hands at the sides. Inhale a deep Yogic breath through both nostrils and at the same time raise the arms slowly up above the head. Hold the breath for one pulse beat, then exhale through the

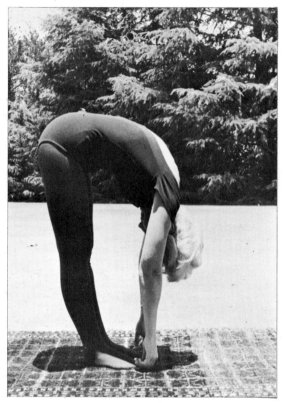

Cleansing Breath.

mouth simultaneously letting the trunk drop forwards from the waist and letting the arms hang down. Then immediately repeat the inhalation and the exhalation in the same manner. You may repeat this exercise up to seven times.

Remarks
When exhaling the breath through the mouth, do so with the prolonged sound of "HA". When it is desired to empty the lungs quickly, it is done by emptying them through the mouth, otherwise we breathe in through the nose and breathe out through the nose.

Concluding Remarks

The value of correct breathing cannot be over-emphasised. There are, of course, many more Pranayama or breathing exercises, but these are the ones most suitable for you to select as daily exercises. There is no necessity to do every breathing exercise every day, but you should make a point of doing the deep Yogic Breath daily, then select the ones you wish to practise and finally finish off the exercises with the Cleansing Breath.

If you practise regularly you will soon feel your whole system responding and you will see the improvement in health reflected in the radiance of your appearance.

Now we shall proceed to learn all about the Yoga Postures, so please read on.

4

The Yoga exercises or postures, or asanas

YOU WILL find on the following pages full details for the performance of the wonderful Yoga postures, including instructions for the correct breathing to be used in combination with them. The practice of these postures will help you to enjoy and maintain radiant health and beauty and will bring a feeling of exhilaration to each and every day.

Accompanying the description of virtually all of the postures is a relative photograph to help you to understand more fully how the exercises are performed. The ages of the pupils who graciously consented to pose for the photographs vary between 40 and 60. They are women living normally active lives as wives, mothers and grandmothers. Some of them are new to Yoga, whilst others are devotees of some years, thus it is obvious that Yoga is not beyond any average woman.

At first you may regard the practice of the postures as a nuisance, but persevere and as you progress you will begin to appreciate their underlying effects, so much so that eventually you will be loath to miss them. You will discover that Yoga is not a brisk daily dozen leaving you tired out and trembling, but instead you will notice that your energies are on the up-and-up and that your body is becoming more vigorous and pliable. You will face all your daily tasks and activities with new enthusiasm, and you will be ready to cope with any unexpected upheavals. You will not tire so easily, either physically or mentally, you will even clock up the walking miles with pleasure as your feet become strengthened.

Once again I would point out that the exercises selected for inclusion here are within reach of all. Some of them are very simple, others are a little more difficult to do, but do not discount the value of the simple postures—even the very advanced Yogis regard the basic postures as an essential part of their routine. If you are unable to complete a posture to your satisfaction, do not lose patience, they will all come to you with a little effort and practice, and you will experience a great sense of achievement when you are able to do with ease something which previously was very uncomfortable. At the same time you will be developing your sense of patience and of perseverance! In the meantime, do what you can because you will benefit from every effort which you make. Start by repeating the exercises only a few times, and then as you become more proficient you can increase the number of repetitions, or, in those cases where it is better to maintain the posture, you will build up and increase the holding period gradually.

As with the Breathing Exercises it is delightful if you are able to do the Yoga postures out-of-doors, preferably first thing in the morning when the air is fresh, but if you cannot do so for any reason then do them indoors in a clean airy room as described previously and at a time to suit yourself.

To refresh your memory, the following points are stressed again:

1. Do not do the exercises immediately after a meal; you should ensure that at least $1\frac{1}{2}$ hours have elapsed after a light meal or $2\frac{1}{2}$ hours after a heavy meal. (This does not apply to the odd exercises which you may wish to do to relieve tensions.)

2. Do not wear any tight clothing. Wear the minimum of under-clothing with tights and a comfortable blouse.

3. Keep a rug or blanket aside for your own personal use as your exercise mat.

4. Do make sure that you will have seclusion, whether indoors or out, and that as far as practicable you will not be disturbed.

5. Do the exercises with sincerity and concentration.

6. The breathing must be combined with the exercises. Make yourself familiar with the deep Yogic Breath before attempting the postures. The deep breathing enriches the blood and as you exercise each particular part of the body, this enriched blood is whipped along by the stimulated circulation and that part which is being exercised receives the benefit of the oxygen-laden blood.

7.   Rest between each posture, and take a relaxing or easy breath between each repetition of the same posture.

Some of the exercises are done whilst seated, some whilst standing, others are done whilst lying down and some are done in the inverted position. The eyes are kept closed whilst performing many of the postures, as in this way you are better able to concentrate. You should direct your attention to whichever part of the body is being exercised by a certain asana. If there are multiple benefits, concentrate on the part of the body which you most wish to improve.

Yoga during pregnancy

If you have never done Yoga before it is not a good idea to start Yoga during pregnancy. On the other hand, if you fall into the category of readers who are already doing Yoga, there will be no need for you to discontinue your practice altogether, although there are certain exercises which you will have to leave out. You must not do any of the abdominal exercises nor any of the inverted postures. You will be able to continue to do the shoulder, neck, eye and leg exercises, the breathing exercises, and, most important of all, the relaxation.

Of the other postures the ones you should concentrate on are:
The Half-Lotus Seat
The Lotus Seat
The Squatting Posture
The Cat Hump
The Bridge
The Dynamic Back Strengthener
The Special Series for Women
The Bust Line Improver

To proceed

The postures have been given English names. This is in accordance with the aim of this book to bring Yoga to you in the most straightforward and lucid manner.

No doubt you are now eager to see what practical Yoga is all about, so with no more ado let us proceed to the wonderful health-giving Yoga postures.

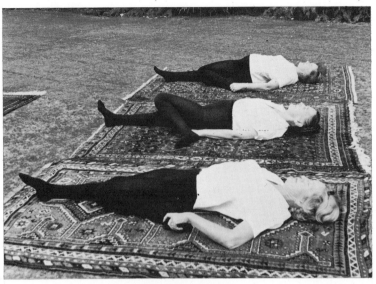

Limbering—Stage 2.

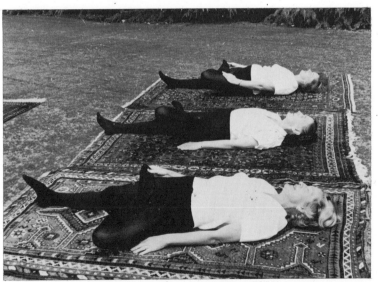

Limbering—Stage 3.

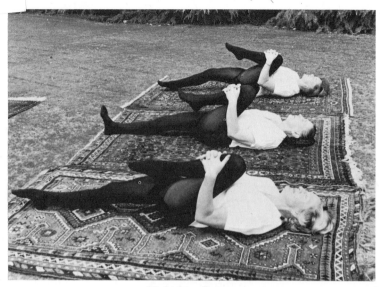

Limbering—Stage 4.

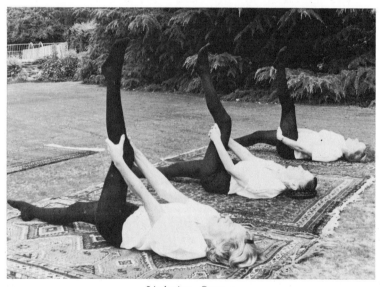

Limbering—Stage 5.

Limbering

Benefits
This exercise will loosen up the body and will help you to sit cross-legged more easily and eventually to sit in the Lotus Seat. It limbers the legs, slims them, loosens the haunches, stretches the ham strings and tones up the sciatic nerves.

Method
1. Lie down flat on the mat, legs extended, feet together and hands at the sides.
2. Each leg is limbered separately, so start by placing the right foot flat on the floor next to the buttocks then take the foot in the right hand and pull the foot and leg around to the outside of the body, so that the heel is close to the thigh, then endeavour to lower the bent leg to the floor. Keep the left leg straight and flat on the floor, and try to keep the buttocks and small of the back down on the mat as well. Now whilst lying in that position, take in three full deep Yogic Breaths, relaxing each time you breathe out. Return the leg to starting position.
3. Remain lying down and place the right foot on the left thigh. Take the right foot in the left hand and pull the heel up as high as possible on to the left thigh, then with the right hand press the right knee down towards the floor. Repeat this movement as often as you wish, then return the leg to starting position.
4. Bend the right knee, clasp it in both hands and pull it on to the chest. Keep the left leg flat on the mat and try to pull the right knee as high up as possible on to the chest. From the clasped knee position, proceed to
5. Straighten the right leg vertically, place the hands behind the knee and pull the leg towards the chest, keeping it straight. Release the hands and lower the leg slowly to the horizontal starting position.

This completes the limbering for the right leg, so now you must repeat the whole exercise with the left leg.

Remarks
After three deep Yogic Breaths in Stage 2, the breathing is

normal. Take a deep breath at the conclusion of the exercise. You will understand the instructions more easily if you will refer to the photographs which reflect each stage of the exercise. It is beneficial to do the limbering before commencing any of the other postures, i.e. at the beginning of your practice.

The Lotus

Some people find the Lotus Seat a very easy position to achieve, others find it almost impossible, especially those with heavy thighs, It is included here because it is an essential part of Yoga and those women who are able to sit in this position should use it. Where

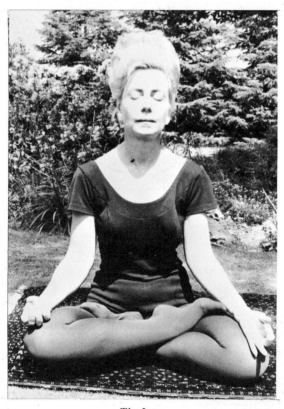

The Lotus.

the Lotus is mentioned and you are unable to sit in the position do not despair because you may sit cross-legged or in the Half-Lotus Seat. At the same time you should continue to limber the legs and keep the Lotus Seat as a goal.

Benefits
This position brings flexibility to the ankles, knees and hips, and is the best position to use whilst carrying out the breathing practices as it keeps the spine erect and enables the newly oxygenated blood to circulate freely to the nervous system. It is also used for the purpose of Meditation, whereby the mind is quietened and rested.

Method
Sit on the mat with both legs extended. Take the right foot in the hands and lift it up as high as possible on the left thigh. Then take the left foot in the hands and slip it over the right leg up on to the right thigh.

Remarks
The knees should be kept down, the back straight, the head up and the shoulders back. The buttocks should be comfortably flat on the floor.

Beware
If you have varicose veins do not sit too long in this position.

The Half-Lotus
This position is easier to attain than the full Lotus and for that reason should be perfected before the Lotus is attempted.

Benefits
This position brings the same benefits as the full Lotus and is used for the same purposes.

Method
Sit on the mat with both legs extended. Take the left foot in the hands and place it with the sole resting on the inside of the right thigh keeping the heel of the left foot as close as possible to the body at the perineum. Then take the right foot and place it in the bend of the left leg.

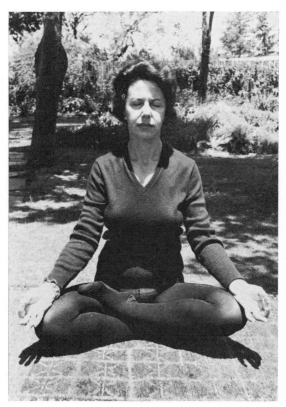

The Half-Lotus.

Remarks

The knees should be kept down, the back straight, the head up and the shoulders back. The buttocks should be comfortably flat on the floor.

The Rolling Ball

Benefits

This exercise is most soothing and if you suffer from insomnia do it before going to bed at night when it will help you to relax and will induce sleep. The Rolling Ball is excellent for limbering the spine, massaging it and keeping it youthful. It brings a supply of newly oxygenated blood to the spine and sympathetic nervous system. As we grow older the spine tends to become rigid and settles in upon itself. This exercise will keep it supple and elongated. "A supple spine is a young spine."

Method
Sit cross-legged on the mat and take the feet in the palms of the hands.
1. Inhale, then bend forward whilst exhaling rapidly through the mouth.
2. Roll backwards onto the spine, (keeping the breath out), taking the legs over the head.
3. Inhale and roll up to sitting position. Maintain the hold upon the feet.

This completes one roll. Repeat the exercise by exhaling rapidly through the mouth whilst bending forward, rolling backwards with empty lungs, inhaling to come up, exhaling to bend forwards and continue in this manner until you have completed up to ten rolls.

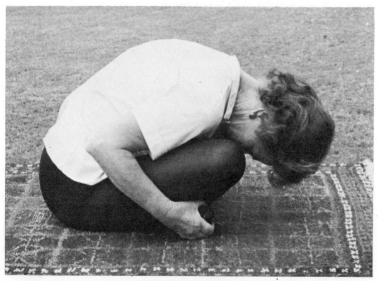

The Rolling Ball—first part.

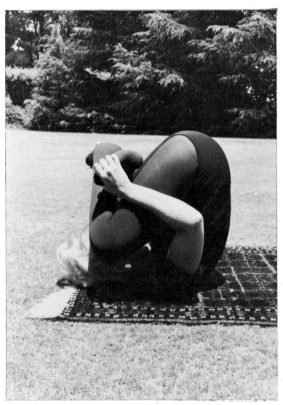

The Rolling Ball—completion of backward roll.

Remarks

Keep the spine rounded when rolling backwards and the chin tucked onto the chest. Make sure that you roll on each vertebra and that you do not fall backwards on a flat back, for if you do you will hurt your back and you will remain there like a beetle unable to roll back to starting position.

Beware

If you have a very hollow back it is advisable to leave this exercise out until you have improved your back by doing the forward spine stretching exercises.

Head and Neck exercises

Almost everyone today complains of pains at the base of the skull and across and between the shoulder blades. This is, in most cases, due to nervous tension and one of the best ways to release this tension is by practising head and neck exercises regularly.

Benefits

All of the exercises given below will help to remove tensions and stiffness from the back of the neck and shoulders. At the same time you will be developing a lovely neck line, and will say goodbye to that double chin!

Head Roll

Sit cross-legged upon the mat, hands resting lightly upon the knees, back straight.

1. Inhale, then holding the breath, drop the chin onto the chest and slowly let the head roll around first to the left, then backwards, then to the right and finally back to starting position. Breathe out.

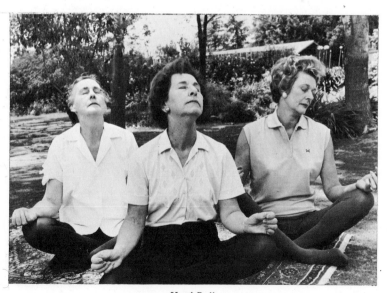

Head Roll.

Repeat the exercise, this time rolling the head first towards the right.

2. Inhale and go through the same movements as in (1) above, but this time take the head around against force.

Head Drop

Place the hands around the neck with the thumbs at the base of the throat. Inhale and drop the head towards the chest, hold the breath and press the head backwards against pressure from the hands; drop the head forwards, press the head backwards, drop the head onto the chest, breathe out and relax.

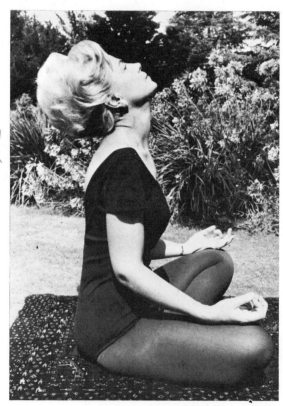

Neck Line Beautifier.

Neck Line Beautifier
Sit with head erect and back straight. Inhale and drop the chin
forwards onto the chest, then hold the breath, raise the head and
drop it backwards. Open the mouth, drop the lower jaw and then
draw it up slowly; drop the jaw, draw it up slowly, and repeat as
often as is comfortable. Return the head to starting position and
exhale.

Head to Shoulder
Sit with the head erect and the back straight. Inhale and take the
head down slowly to the left shoulder trying to place the left ear

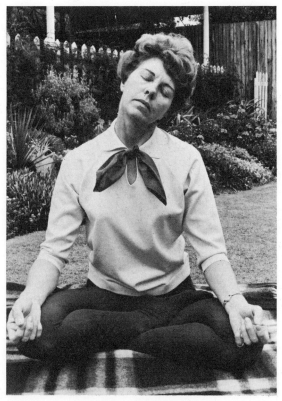

Head to Shoulder.

on the left shoulder; exhale and return to starting position. Inhale and move the head slowly down to the right shoulder, trying to place the right ear on the right shoulder.

Exhale and return to starting position.

Remarks

It is important in this exercise that the shoulders do not move. Do not bring the shoulders up to the ears, but take the ears down to the shoulders. DO NOT STRAIN, or you will have a stiff neck!

Neck massage

Finish the exercises by massaging the back of the neck. This is done by placing the fingers at the base of the skull and then moving them firmly up into the hairline and then down into the neck and down the upper portion of the spine. Repeat this movement frequently and then knead down the spine with the cushions of the finger tips, and up the spine again into the hair line. This will make the whole of the neck and shoulder area feel warm and relaxed.

Remarks

All of the above exercises can be done whilst sitting upright in a chair, and can be repeated as often as desired. They are not strenuous exercises, so can be done at any time it is convenient to you—perhaps whilst you are taking your bath?

Eye exercises

The eyes are the windows of the soul! They reflect our personalities and also the state of our health. Eyes should never be neglected and they deserve the best possible attention. A little time devoted to exercising the eyes every day can strengthen and beautify them. There are always a few idle moments during the day when the following exercises can be done.

Benefits

If you do the exercises regularly they will strengthen the eyes, particularly if they are followed by "palming". Palming is done by rubbing the hands together then closing your eyes and covering them with the palms, placing the right hand over the left hand.

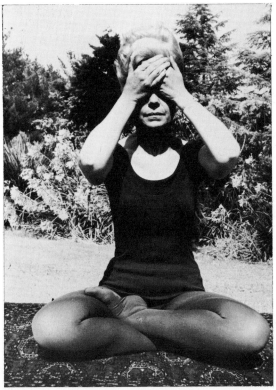

Eye exercises—palming.

Method

Here again the exercises can be done sitting in a chair, or even whilst sitting in a car. Breathe normally and repeat each of the exercises five times and remember to blink the eyes after completing each exercise. DO NOT MOVE THE HEAD, BUT ONLY THE EYES.

1. Keep the head erect and look straight in front of you, then fix the gaze upon the tip of the nose. Repeat.
2. Keep the head erect, then lift the eyes and gaze to the upper left corner, then down to the lower right corner. Repeat.
3. Keep the head erect, then lift the eyes up to the right corner, and then down to the lower left corner. Repeat.

4. Look straight in front of you and then swing the eyes from left to right, horizontally. Repeat.
5. Look straight in front of you, then look downwards and then roll the eyes around, first clockwise and then anticlockwise. Repeat.

Remarks

Remember to blink between each exercise and finish off the series by palming. Naturally, you will not do the exercises whilst actually driving!

Ankle Rotation and Foot Stretch

Benefits

We cannot have happy faces with unhappy feet! Most feet are very badly treated, but are expected to render their owners efficient service for a very long time. The Ankle Rotation and Foot Stretch will keep the ankles trim, will strengthen the arches and loosen up the toes.

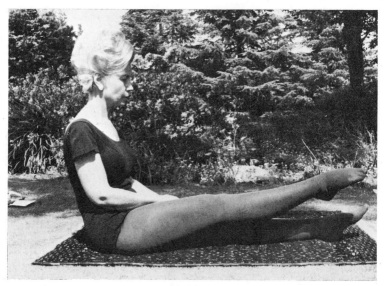

Ankle Rotation.

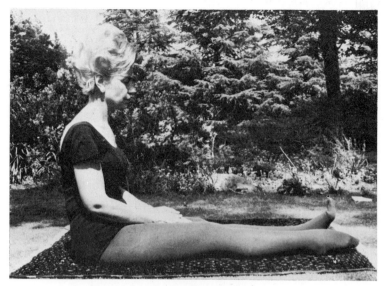

Foot Stretch.

Method

1. Sit on the floor, stretch out the legs with the feet together, and have the hands resting lightly upon the lap. Raise the right leg six inches from the floor and slowly rotate the ankle clockwise approximately ten times, then anti-clockwise approximately ten times, then lower the leg to the floor. Repeat the exercise with the left leg.

2. Keep the feet together and slowly stretch the feet and toes downwards towards the mat, then slowly stretch the feet and toes upwards, separate the toes and maintain the upward stretch for a few seconds, then stretch the feet down towards the floor again, then up, and so on. Repeat approximately five times.

Remarks

Before you rise in the morning make it a habit to stretch the body. First a complete stretch with legs and arms, and then stretch each leg alternately. Stretch down with the heels and not with the toes.

The Stretches

Benefits

Stretch for beauty! Remember that one of the aims of Yoga is to keep the body supple so the Stretches should be done every day. They are simple but their benefits are multiple and they do, in fact, stretch the whole of the trunk with particular emphasis on the all-important spine and the rib cage. They slim the waist and the abdomen, increase the capacity of and strengthen the lungs, and keep the spine supple and youthful.

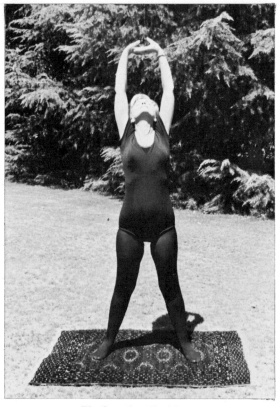

The Stretches—Position 2.

Method

1. *Starting Position* Stand erect, feet about eighteen inches apart, hands at the sides.

2. *Overhead Stretch* Inhale as you slowly raise the arms sideways behind the line of the shoulders until they are right above the head, then interlock the fingers and turn the palms upwards and stretch right up with the trunk and arms— s-t-r-e-t-c-h, then lower the arms sideways whilst exhaling and bringing them down behind the line of the shoulders back to starting position. Relax by taking in a deep Yogic Breath and then repeat the overhead stretch once more.

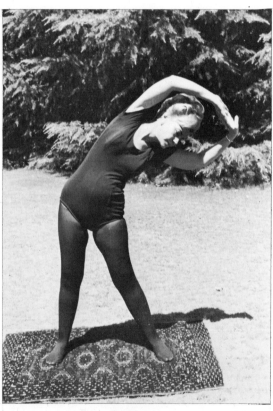

Position 3.

3. *Sideways Stretch*   Inhale whilst stretching upwards as in (2), interlock the fingers and then using the arms to frame the head, slowly bend the trunk to the left, then to the right, (retaining the breath whilst bending), then return to the upright position and exhale whilst lowering the arms to starting position. Take in a deep Yogic Breath, and then repeat the Sideways Stretch once more.

4. *Forward and Backward Stretch*   Inhale whilst stretching upwards in the same manner as before, then slowly stretch the trunk forwards keeping the arms and head up, then stretch

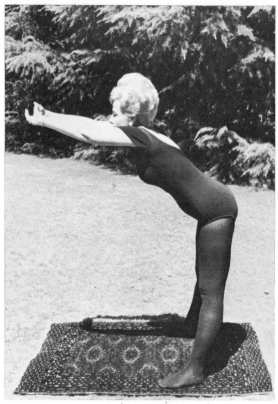

Position 4. Forward.

backwards, return to the upright position, then exhale whilst slowly returning to starting position. Take in a deep Yogic Breath, and then repeat the Forward and Backward Stretch once more.

5. *All The Way Around Stretch* Inhale whilst stretching upwards as before, then bend the trunk slightly forward and keeping the arms up and swivelling within the hips, make a circle by moving slowly round to the left, backwards, to the right, to the centre, and then straighten to the upright position. Exhale whilst lowering the arms and return to starting position.

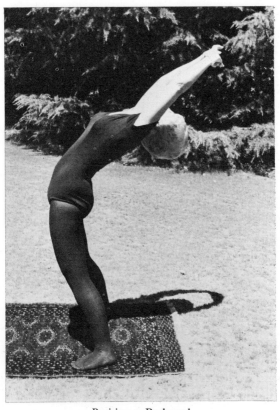

Position 4. Backward.

Take in a deep Yogic Breath, and then repeat the Stretch by circling in the opposite direction, i.e. right, back, left, centre, up, and back to starting position.

Remarks

These Stretches are best done in the morning upon arising. Do them before an open window.

Shoulder exercises

Benefits

All of the shoulder exercises will help to relieve tensions across the shoulders and between the shoulder blades. Nervous tension causes nagging pains at the base of the skull and between and across the shoulders. Learn to relax mentally and physically, and use the shoulder exercises to loosen up the shoulders and back. The exercises are invaluable for anyone suffering from neuritis and also for anyone who spends long hours over an office desk or machine of any kind.

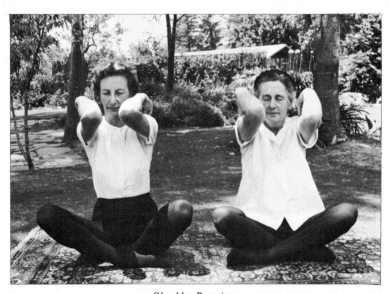

Shoulder Rotation.

Shoulder Rotation

Method

Sit cross-legged or in the Lotus Seat upon the mat. Place the hands upon the shoulders, elbows tucked into the sides. Inhale and then rotate the elbows slowly backwards approximately three times and then change the direction of the elbows and rotate them slowly forwards three times. Exhale and rest. Repeat as often as desired.

Remarks

The exercise must be done slowly and deliberately and with the endeavour to make the shoulder blades meet at the back.

Shoulder Shrugs

Method

Sit cross-legged or in the Lotus Seat upon the mat and rest the hands on the knees. Breathe normally and shrug the right shoulder up and down approximately ten times; then shrug the left shoulder in the same way for the same number of times, and finally shrug both shoulders together.

Remarks

This exercise also strengthens the pectoral muscles so the bosom receives an uplift!

Swimming

Method

1. Stand erect, feet together, hands at the sides.
2. Breathe normally and then slowly rotate the right shoulder backwards and round, almost in the same way as when swimming backstroke, but keeping the hands at the sides. Repeat the movement ten times.
3. Rotate the left shoulder in the same manner, and repeat the movement the same number of times.
4. Rotate both shoulders at the same time, endeavouring to make the shoulder blades meet at the back. Repeat ten times.
5. Relax, and then go through the whole exercise again, but this time rotate the shoulders forward and round, as in overarm swimming.

Remarks

The Shoulder Exercises, like the Head and Neck Exercises, can be done at any time to suit yourself. Try to become conscious of exercise, so that when you have a spare moment and, for example, you feel tiredness across the shoulders, do the shoulder exercises. They can be done at the office or in the workroom, and the shoulder shrugs can be done whilst driving.

Use your exercises and make them work for you—don't keep them in cotton wool, bring them out and use them.

You can do the exercises whilst sitting on a chair.

Wide Angle Stretch—standing

Benefits

This exercise strengthens and stretches the muscles of the legs and spine, thus keeping them youthful and firm. The muscles on the inside of the legs are the first muscles of the legs to go lax. Practise this exercise regularly and you need never be afraid to appear in a

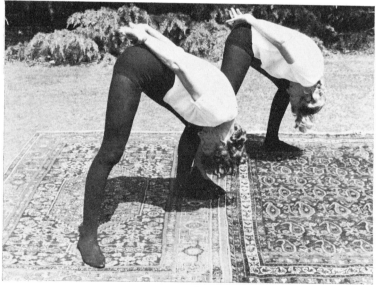

Wide Angle Stretch—standing.

bathing suit! As the head is brought down to the ankle, the brain receives a flow of blood and the muscles and tissues of the face are fed, thus keeping wrinkles at bay.

Method
1. Stand erect and part the legs as wide as possible. Clasp the hands behind the back.
2. Inhale, then exhale as you bend the trunk over towards the inside of the right leg, at the same time bending the right knee and trying to take the head down to the inside of the right ankle. Hold the position for a few seconds.
3. Inhale and slowly push yourself up to position (1), using the muscles of the legs.
4. Exhale and repeat the exercise by bending over to the inside of the left ankle. Hold the position for a few seconds, then
5. Inhale and return to position (1) and continue with the exercise.

Repeat the complete exercise as often as is comfortable.

Remarks
Bend from the hips and not from the waist.

Trunk Backward Bend

Benefits
This posture, although simple, has many benefits. It will reduce the fat on the abdomen and strengthen and firm the thighs. It improves the line of the throat, strengthens the backbone and stimulates the adrenals or "action" glands.

Method
1. Stand erect, place the feet together and the hands across the small of the back, thumbs to the front of the body.
2. Inhale and slowly bend the trunk backwards, then exhale and return to position (1).
3. Take a deep Yogic Breath and then repeat the exercise as often as is comfortable.

Remarks
Endeavour to get the bend in the small of the back.

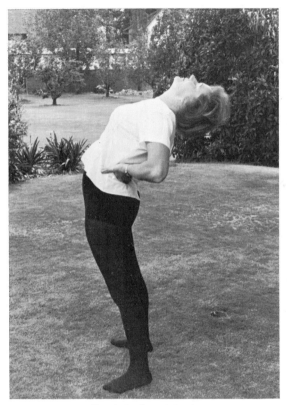

Trunk Backward Bend.

Standing Siamese posture

Benefits

This is an exercise which will help to give you that slim waistline so desired by every woman, and "spare tyres" will disappear. It will expand the rib cage, thus increasing the lung capacity and strengthening the lungs, whilst it also tones the spine.

Method

1. Stand erect with the feet apart. Place the right hand on top of the head and turn the gaze to the inside of the right elbow.

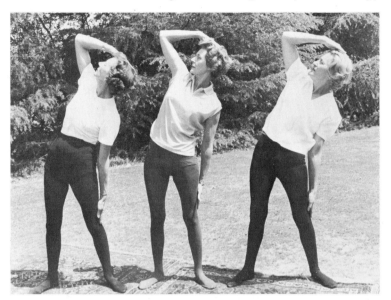

Standing Siamese posture.

Keep the left arm at the left side. Inhale, then exhale as you bend the trunk to the left, sliding the left arm down the left leg as far as you are able to, then inhale and return to starting position. Exhale and repeat the sideways bend. Repeat the exercise as often as is comfortable.

2. Place the left hand on top of the head and turn the gaze to the inside of the left elbow. Keep the right arm at the right side. Inhale, then exhale as you bend the trunk to the right, sliding the right arm down the right leg as far as you are able to, then inhale while returning to starting position. Exhale and repeat the sideways bend.

    Repeat the bend to the right the same number of times that you bent to the left.

Remarks

This is a SIDEWAYS bend, not a FORWARD bend, so do not make the mistake of bending the trunk forwards.

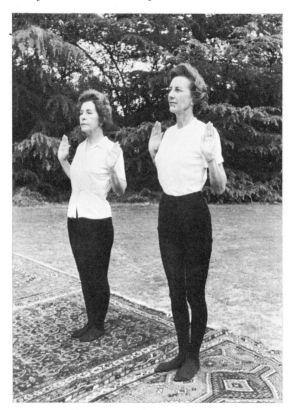

Chest and Arm Stretch—position 1.

Chest and Arm Stretch

Benefits

Here is another exercise for relieving the tensions and pains across the shoulders. It also stretches the ham strings in the legs, reduces fat on the abdomen and the upper arms, and brings the blood to the brain and helps eliminate wrinkles. All the forward bending exercises also help to condition the hair.

Method

Stand erect with the feet together, hands at the sides.

1.   Inhale and draw the hands up to the shoulders.

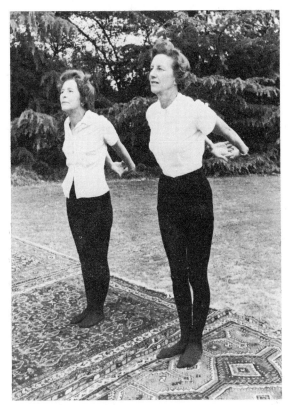

Position 3.

2. Exhale and stretch the arms out horizontally in front of the shoulders.
3. Inhale and turn the hands to the outside of the body and take the arms right around to the back and clasp the hands whilst keeping the arms up.
4. Exhale and bend backwards from the waist. Maintain this position for a few seconds, then inhale and return to standing position.
5. Exhale and still keeping the arms up, bend forward with the trunk and let the head hang down. Maintain this position for a few seconds, inhale and raise the trunk to the upright

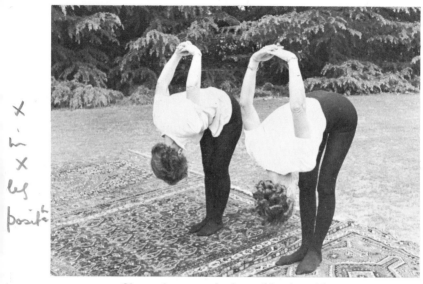

Chest and arm stretch—forward bend, position 5.

position still keeping the arms up, then exhale and return to starting position with the hands at the sides.

Take a deep Yogic Breath and then repeat the exercise as often as is comfortable, pausing between each repetition in order to relax with a deep breath.

Remarks

The exercise sounds complicated, but it is not. It is easier in this case to have someone read out the instructions to you as you are doing the exercise. The arms must not be allowed to drop. They must remain in the raised position for the entire exercise. Always remember to take a deep Yogic Breath between the repetitions of all of the exercises. Do not strain.

The Eagle

Benefits

This posture helps us to retain and improve our sense of balance and it also teaches us concentration. It will keep the ovaries functioning properly and will strengthen the leg muscles.

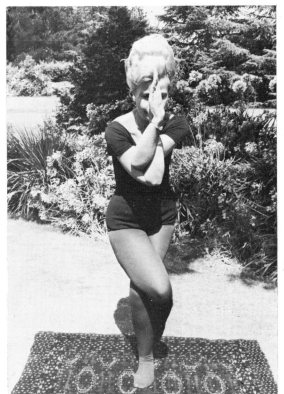

The Eagle—front view.

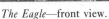

Method

Stand erect with the feet together. Bend the left knee slightly and wrap the right leg around the left leg bringing the toes of the right leg to the inside of the ankle of the left leg. Place the right arm underneath the left arm, and then place the palms of the hands together. Sink down slightly on the haunches and place the clasped hands in front of the face. Maintain the position for as long as is comfortable whilst breathing easily. Slowly unwind the position and take a deep Yogic Breath. Repeat the exercise by wrapping the left leg around the right leg, and by placing the left arm underneath the right arm, and maintaining the final position for as long

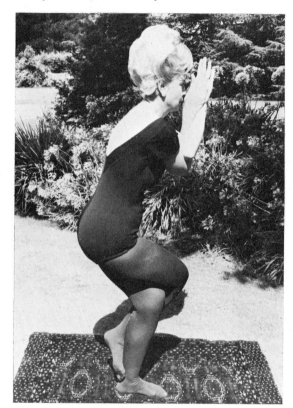

Side view.

as is comfortable whilst breathing easily. Unwind slowly and relax.

Remarks
This is one of the exercises where it is necessary to hold the posture, rather than repeat it. Start by holding it for a short while and slowly build up the holding time as you progress with Yoga. It helps to maintain the balance whilst holding the posture to fix the eyes on a selected spot and to keep the gaze fixed on that spot until you relax the position.

Toe Balance

Benefits

The Toe Balance strengthens the arches of the feet and the legs. It also improves our sense of balance and our powers of concentration.

Method

Stand erect, feet together, hands on the hips. Place the right foot behind the left ankle, then inhale and raise up onto the left foot and endeavour to maintain the position for a few seconds. Exhale and return to starting position.

Repeat the exercise with the other foot.

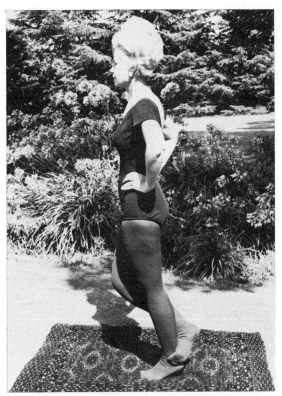

The Toe Balance—side view.

Remarks

The exercise is a simple one, but it is remarkably difficult to maintain the balance, so do not despair if you cannot do it the first time you try. It will take quite a while to perfect this exercise, and you may repeat it as often as you wish. The toes are probably the least exercised parts of the body. The Toe Balance will keep them supple.

The Jack Knife

Benefits

Two of the secrets of eternal youth are a supple spine and youthful knees. The "Jack Knife" posture will rejuvenate and strengthen

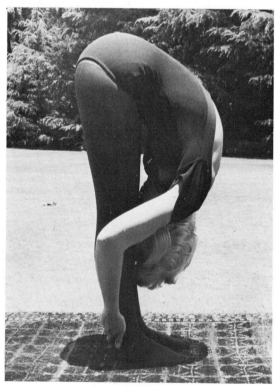

The Jack-knife.

your spine and put "spring" into your legs and knees. It will take excess fat off the abdomen, feed the brain and facial tissues, reduce wrinkles, and keep sciatica at bay. It will also improve the health of the hair.

Method
1. Stand erect with the feet together, hands at the sides.
2. Inhale, then bend forward from the hips whilst exhaling and sliding the hands down the back of the legs. Clasp the ankles and pull the head down onto the knees. Maintain the position with the breath out for a few seconds.
3. Inhale and slowly straighten up to position (1).

   Take a deep Yogic Breath and then repeat the exercise. The posture may be repeated three times at the beginning but as you advance and gain experience in the practice of Yoga you may repeat the posture as many times as is comfortable.

Remarks
Do not bend from the waist, but bend from the hips, and do not jerk. If you are unable to take the head down to the knees take it down just as far as is comfortable, but do not bend the knees. Let the head drop downwards, do not keep it raised.

The Stork

Benefits
As we grow older we tend to lose our sense of balance. This posture will improve it and will also teach us concentration. It will also strengthen the legs.

Method
Stand erect, feet together. Place the right leg high up on the thigh of the left leg and then drop the knee. Clasp the hands and extend the hands and arms above the head. Fix the eyes on one particular spot, breathe easily and maintain the posture for as long as you can.

   Relax, change legs and repeat the posture.

Remarks
This posture must be held and not repeated, therefore try to build up the time you are able to maintain it.

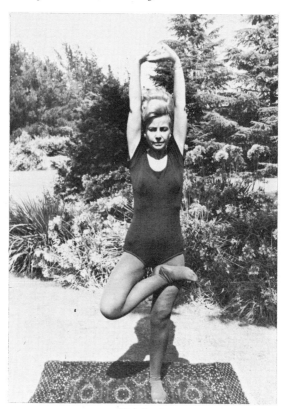

The Stork.

The Stomach Lift

If you suffer from constipation, or have excess fat on the stomach, then this is the exercise for you.

Benefits

One of the best exercises for strengthening the muscles of the abdomen and ridding it of fat. Tones up all the internal organs and is marvellous for stimulating the bowels. If you are suffering from menopausal or menstrual disorders, prolapse or sterility, regular practice of the Stomach Lift will render a definite improvement in your condition.

Method

Stand erect with the feet about eighteen inches apart. Inhale, then exhale and make sure the lungs are completely empty, rest your hands on your upper thighs, bend your knees slightly, tip the trunk slightly forward, arch the back, secure the chin on to the chest, pull the stomach in towards the backbone and then draw it up underneath the ribs and maintain the position for as long as you can. Relax the position and inhale, take a deep Yogic Breath and then repeat the exercise four to six times.

Remarks

This exercise should never be done unless the stomach is empty,

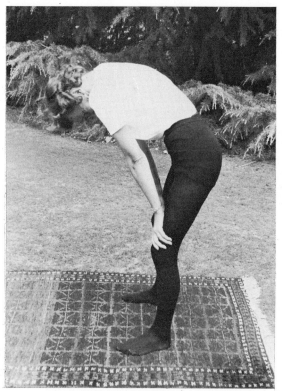

The Stomach Lift.

therefore it is best to do it first thing in the morning upon arising. If it is done during the day, be sure that at least $1\frac{1}{2}$ hours have elapsed after a light meal, or $2\frac{1}{2}$ hours after a heavier one. When the stomach is lifted there should be a hollow underneath the ribs and the abdomen should be concave. Do not do the exercise whilst menstruating.

Bust Line Improver
This is not strictly a YOGA exercise, but it is one which should be practised by all women.

Benefits
Although the exercise is simple it is most beneficial in keeping the pectoral muscles toned. These muscles keep the "uplift" in the bosom.

Method
Sit cross-legged on the mat, or you may sit upright in a chair. Fold the arms and clasp the upper forearms near the elbows with the opposite hand. Raise the arms outwards and then push with

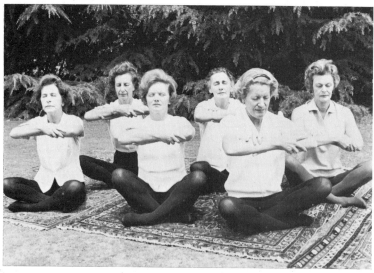

Bust Line Improver.

the hands firmly towards the elbows. Repeat the short pushing movements as often as possible, and then change the position of the hands, i.e. if you have had the right hand on the inside of the left arm and the left hand on the outside of the right arm, change around so that the left hand is on the inside of the right arm and the right hand on the outside of the left arm. Repeat the exercise as often as possible.

Remarks
Make it a habit to do this exercise every day, and if you make it part of your bath routine you will not forget to do it.

Special Series for Women

Benefits
This series of exercises if practised regularly will benefit very considerably those women who suffer from various problems related to the reproductive organs. They will tone up the internal organs, will delay menopause, stop flooding, and at the same time they will also strengthen the back.

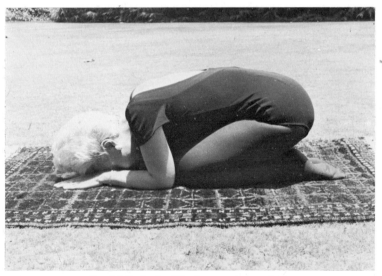

Special Series for Women—starting position.

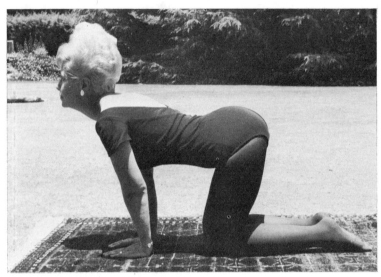

Special Series for Women—position 2.

Method

1. Kneel down and sit on the heels. Place the forearms parallel on the floor and have the elbows touching the knees.
2. Inhale, straighten the arms and come up on to the knees whilst dropping the abdomen and making a saddle back and raising the head upwards and backwards.
3. Exhale, lower the arms and head and place the head between the arms, the nose between the knees and keep the buttocks in the raised position.
4. Inhale and take the Cat Hump position, straightening the arms and drawing the abdomen in and up and tucking the chin onto the chest.
5. Exhale and return to starting position.

Repeat the exercise up to ten times, keeping the movements smooth and continuous.

Remarks

This exercise can be done during pregnancy, but needless to say you will first obtain your doctor's permission before attempting this or any other exercises during pregnancy.

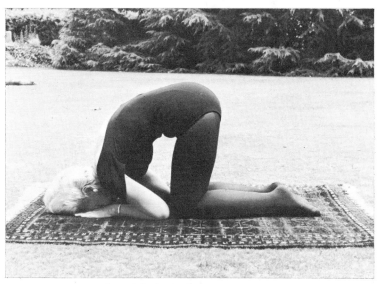

Special Series for Women—position 3.

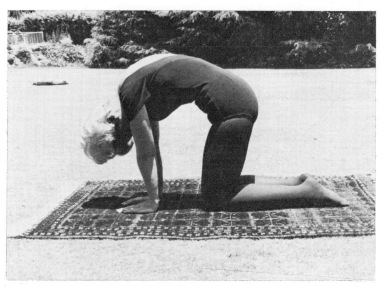

Special Series for Women—position 4.

Anti-Wrinkle exercise

Benefits

There will be no need for you to visit the beauty parlour for a facial! This exercise will fill out lines and wrinkles and tone up the skin of the face.

Method

Sit cross-legged on the mat and close the fingers of each hand around the thumbs. Press hard on the thumbs and place the hands behind the back, right fist over the left fist. Inhale, then hold the breath and bend over to the left knee. Hold the breath and the

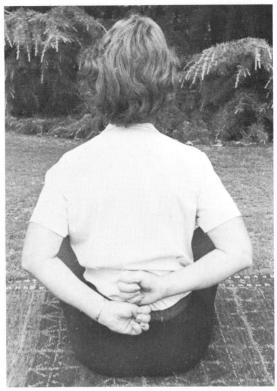

Anti-Wrinkle exercise—first position.

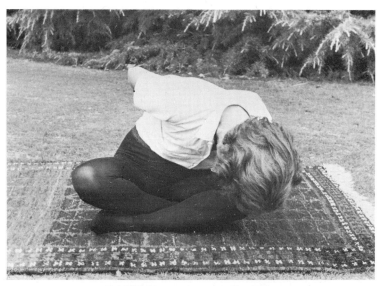

Anti-Wrinkle exercise—second position.

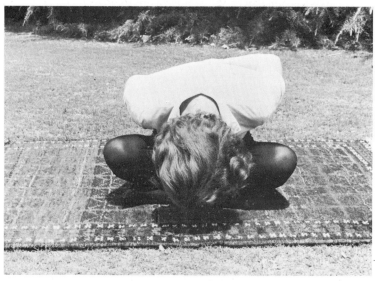

Anti-Wrinkle exercise—completed.

position for as long as possible, then exhale and return to starting position. Inhale and repeat the exercise to the right knee, exhale to return to starting position, then inhale and bend forward towards the mat in the central position. Maintain the position for as long as comfortable, then exhale and return to starting position. These three movements make up the entire exercise. You may repeat the exercise as often as comfortable.

Remarks
As women grow older the circulation in the face tends to lessen and this is one of the causes of wrinkles. Feeding the tissues will help to keep the skin blooming and smooth and the complexion radiant. Naturally you must also ensure that you eat the right foods.

Beware
If you suffer from high blood pressure do not do this exercise.

The Squatting posture

Benefits
This exercise is beneficial to all those suffering from constipation. It will tighten and strengthen the muscles of the vagina and anus and help where there are haemorrhoids. The tendons at the back of the legs are stretched.

Method
Keep the feet parallel and flat on the floor and about 2 inches apart. Squat down on the haunches, keeping the feet flat on the floor and extend the arms and clasp the hands. Inhale, then exhale, and draw up all the muscles of the anus and the vagina—hold the breath out and maintain the position for a few seconds, then inhale and relax.

Repeat the exercise as often as is comfortable, but be careful when relaxing the contraction that you do not let go with force.

Remarks
If it is not possible to squat down with the feet flat on the floor without toppling over, then hold on to the end of the bed or something which is firm until you have stretched the muscles down the back of the calves, and are able to do the exercise with

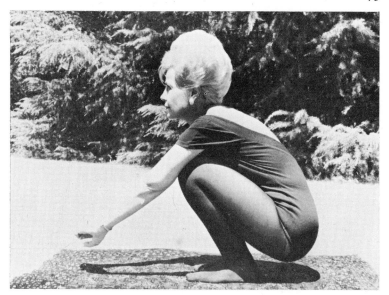

Squatting posture.

ease. This exercise can be done during pregnancy, with your doctor's permission.

Cat Hump

Benefits
This exercise has an important effect on women's internal organs, massaging and toning them, and at the same time it keeps the spine flexible.

Method
Kneel down on the mat on the hands and knees, keeping the arms straight and letting the head hang downwards. Inhale and let the abdomen drop downwards whilst assuming a "saddle-back" position, raising the head and tilting the end of the spine upwards; exhale and arch the back, drawing in the abdomen and tucking in the buttocks. Inhale and assume the saddle-back position, exhale and arch the back, and continue with the exercise in this manner. You may repeat the exercise as often as comfortable.

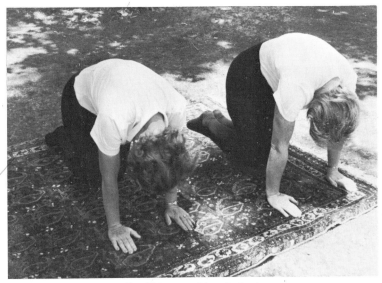

Cat Hump—arching the back.

Remarks

Whilst drawing in the abdomen and tucking in the buttocks, also tighten the muscles of the anus and the vagina. This exercise can be done during pregnancy, with your doctor's permission.

The Tortoise

Usually most people associate Yoga with standing on one's head! However, there is no need for the mature woman to feel that she has to stand on her head in order to justify common belief. Indeed, it would be foolish for the average older woman who has led a sedentary life to attempt head stands. With the following exercise and with the practice of the Shoulder Stand you may enjoy the benefits of the Head Stand without any of its disadvantages.

What is more, the following exercise even helps the toes to remain supple!

Benefits

The Tortoise helps to bring the blood to the brain and feeds it with the newly enriched supply. The Pineal and Pituitary glands

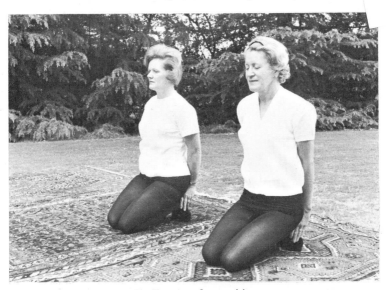

The Tortoise—first position.

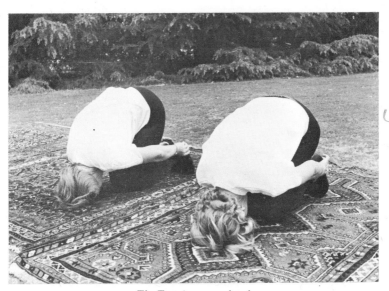

The Tortoise—completed.

are benefited, the sinuses are cleared and the tissues of the face are fed. The eyes and the ears are benefited and Migraine will respond.

Method

Kneel down on the mat with the toes inverted, then sit back on the heels and clasp them with the fingers. Inhale, then exhale and whilst retaining the grip on the heels bend forward with the trunk and raise the buttocks and roll over on to the top of the head. Keep the feet on the floor and maintain the position for a few seconds, then inhale, raise the trunk and sit back on the heels once again.

The exercise may be repeated as often as is comfortable.

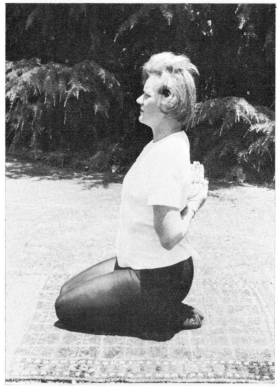

Anti-Asthma exercise—first part.

Anti-Asthma exercise

Benefits
This exercise helps asthmatic sufferers. It also clears the sinuses and at the same time brings the blood to the head and brain and helps to smooth out wrinkles. One of the aims of Yoga is to keep the arteries in an elastic condition, and another is to stimulate the circulation. The heart has a busy time pumping the blood up to the head so this exercise will help the heart with its work.

Method
Sit down on the mat on the knees, put the hands behind the back and place the palms together, thumbs next to the spine. Inhale whilst bending forward and putting the nose between the knees, pause, then exhale and return to starting position. Inhale, exhale whilst bending forward and putting the nose between the knees, pause, then inhale and come up. Repeat the exercise as often as desired.

Remarks
Keep the shoulders well back whilst doing the exercise, and note

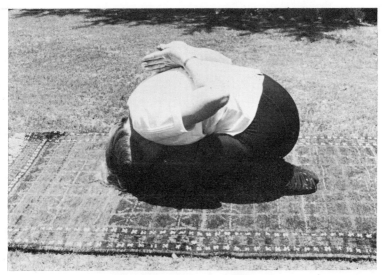

Anti-Asthma exercise—completed.

particularly that whilst bending forward you do so first on an inhalation and then the following time on an exhalation. This pattern is repeated throughout the exercise.

The exercise may also be done with the fingers pointing upwards towards the shoulders, thumbs to the outside, as in the photograph.

The Swan

Benefits
This exercise has a delightful rhythm about it, and gently stretches the spine and trunk. It has a most beneficial effect on the liver, kidney and adrenals, will reduce fat on the abdomen and will keep your knees youthful! The internal organs are massaged and elimination is improved.

Method
1. Lie down on the abdomen and place the hands palms down underneath the shoulders, keep the feet together and invert the toes.

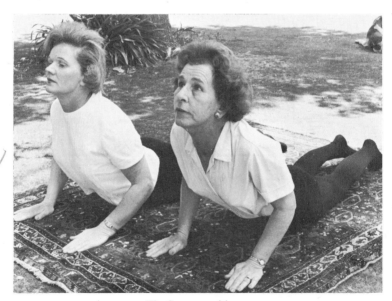

The Swan—position 2.

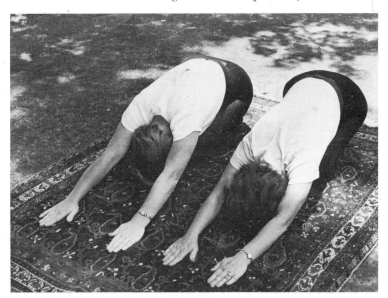

The Swan—position 3.

2. Inhale and then push up with the arms and raise your head, shoulders and abdomen until the arms are straight and there is pressure in the small of the back, i.e. where the spine begins to curve upwards from the buttocks.

3. Exhale and sit back on the heels whilst keeping the palms on the floor and placing the forehead on the mat. The palms should not move, the stretching movement should all take place in the body.

4. Inhale and raise the buttocks and keeping the same rhythmic movement slide the body forward until once again the arms are straight and the lower part of the body is on the floor with the head, shoulders, chest and abdomen raised and being supported by the hands and arms.

5. Exhale and sink to starting position.

You may do the exercise continuously, or you may take an easy breath and rest between each repetition, and you may repeat the exercise as often as is comfortable.

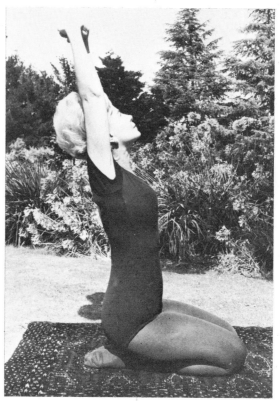

Sideways Slip—starting position.

Sideways Slip posture

Benefits

Reduces the hips, thighs and waistline. Massages kidneys and colon, and stimulates evacuation.

Method

Sit down on the heels, keeping the legs together.

1. Inhale and raise the arms above the head, clasp the hands and at the same time come up onto the knees.
2. Exhale and swing the arms over to the right and sit down to the left of the bent legs.

3. Inhale and raise the body and arms and stretch up onto the knees.
4. Exhale and swing the arms to the left and sit down to the right of the bent legs.
5. Inhale and come up onto the knees stretching the arms up above the head.
6. Sink down onto the heels whilst exhaling.
   Repeat the exercise as often as is desired.

Remarks
When raising the trunk and stretching up onto the knees do not

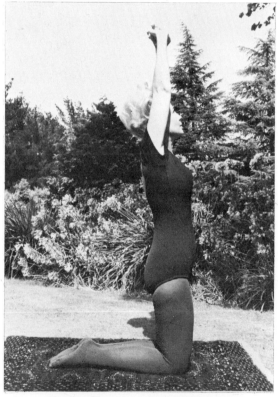

Sideways Slip—stretching up onto knees.

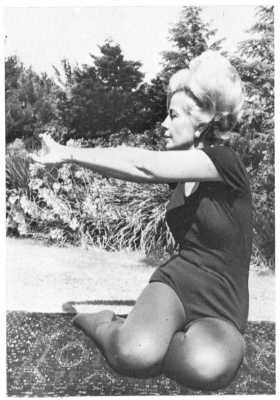

Sideways Slip—swinging arms to side.

bend forward with the trunk in order to scoop yourself up, but keep the spine erect and push upwards with the thighs. This is a most graceful exercise when well done.

The Rabbit

Benefits
The forward stretching of the trunk massages all of the internal organs, and is particularly beneficial to the liver. The rib cage is stretched, elimination is improved, and the thighs are reduced. The knees, ankles and insteps are strengthened.

Method

1. Kneel down on the mat, then sit back on the heels, raise the arms up above the head and keep them close to the ears and place the palms of the hands together.

2. Inhale, then exhale whilst lowering the trunk and arms to the floor, keeping the buttocks on the heels. Place the nose between the knees and then stretch out with the trunk and the arms as far as possible along the floor. Maintain the posture for a few seconds, then

3. Inhale whilst raising the arms and trunk back to starting

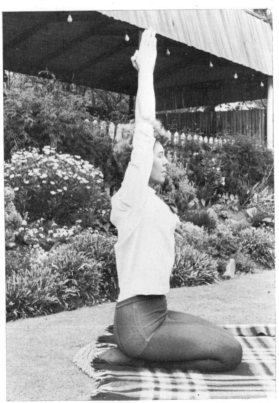

The Rabbit—starting position.

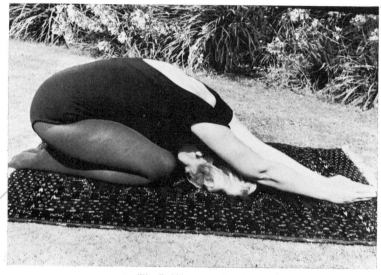

The Rabbit—completed.

position, i.e. sitting on the heels, then sway backwards, exhale whilst bending forwards and repeat the exercise as often as is wished.

Remarks
Really try to get the trunk to move when you stretch forwards.

Dynamic Back Strengthener
This exercise only takes ten seconds to do.

Benefits
The muscles of the back are strengthened, and those of the vagina and anus are toned.

Method
Lie down on the back, hands stretched up above the head, feet placed flat on the floor next to the buttocks. Inhale and then press the small of the back down to the mat, at the same time tightening the buttocks and drawing up the orifices of the body. Hold the breath and maintain the posture for a count of ten, then exhale and relax and return to starting position.

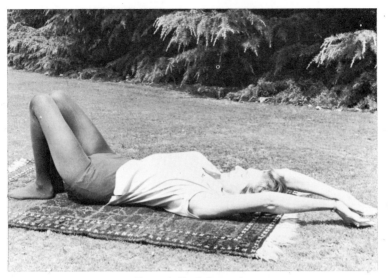

Dynamic Back Strengthener.

Remarks

This posture only needs to be done once per day. This exercise can be done during pregnancy, but keep the hands and arms at the sides.

Back Strengthening posture

Benefits

This posture strengthens the back and abdominal muscles, and will relieve constipation.

Method

Lie down on the mat with the hands clasped behind the head and the legs stretched out and together. Inhale and slowly raise the head, arms, hands and shoulders from the floor whilst simultaneously raising both legs to an angle of 45°, keeping the back flat upon the floor. Hold the breath and hold the position for as long as possible, then exhale and slowly lower the head, arms and legs and return to starting position.

Take a deep relaxing Yogic Breath and then repeat the exercise. The exercise may be repeated up to five times.

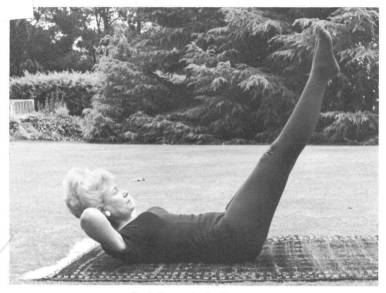

Back Strengthening Posture.

The Bridge (or arch)

Benefits
This posture will assist prolapse and will strengthen the internal organs and weak back muscles.

Method
Lie down on the back on the mat, hands at the sides, palms down, and place the feet together close to the buttocks. Inhale and raise the body, keeping the shoulders, the head and the feet on the floor, and form an arch or a bridge with the body. Easy breathe and maintain the position for as long as comfortable, then inhale, exhale, and slowly return to starting position.

Take a deep relaxing breath and repeat the exercise up to five times.

Remarks
This exercise may be done during pregnancy, with your doctor's permission.

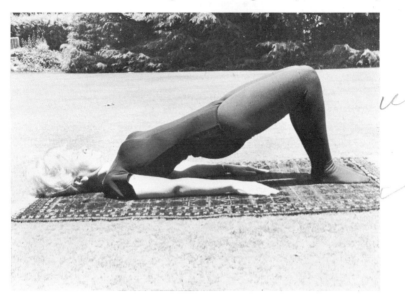

The Bridge (or arch).

Reducing posture

This is one posture a great many readers will have been waiting for!

Benefits

This is an over-all reducing posture. The longer the posture is held the more beneficial it will be. Excess fat on tummies will positively melt away.

Method

Lie down flat on the back on the mat, hands at the sides with the palms resting against the thighs, feet together, legs stretched out. Inhale and raise the head and shoulders and the legs about 6 inches from the floor. Bend the knees slightly so that the calves are parallel with the floor. Easy breathe in this position and hold it for as long as you can, then inhale, exhale, and slowly return to starting position.

Take a deep Yogic Breath and repeat the posture as often as is comfortable.

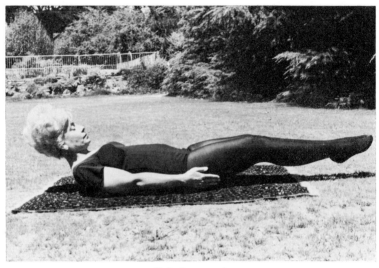

Reducing posture.

Remarks

Endeavour to build up the time that you are able to hold the posture, as it is more beneficial to hold it rather than to keep repeating it.

Wide Angle Posture—sitting

Benefits

This exercise is particularly good for the lumbar region of the back. It also stimulates the bowels and tones up the muscles on the inside of the upper leg. The sciatic nerves are stretched and the arms are firmed.

Method

Sit on the mat and stretch the legs as far apart as possible. Clasp the hands and rest them upon the left knee. Inhale, exhale, pull in the abdominal muscles, lift the trunk and stretch over towards the left foot, endeavouring to clasp the left instep and to place the elbows down on either side of the left knee. Hold the posture for a few seconds, then release the hands, inhale and return to starting position.

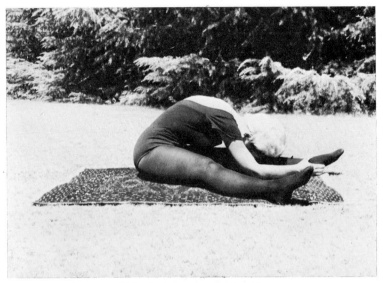

Wide Angle posture—to the side.

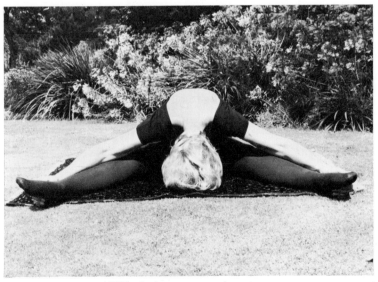

Wide Angle posture—to the centre.

Repeat with the right leg.

Take a deep relaxing breath at the conclusion of the exercise and then repeat as often as comfortable.

Remarks

Endeavour to keep the legs straight. If it is not possible to clasp the instep, then bend only as far as you can without strain and rest the hands on the leg. Do not jerk whilst doing this exercise— it must be done slowly and purposefully.

Keep the buttocks flat upon the floor.

When you are able to stretch to the side with ease, then endeavour to take the head down to the mat in the centre between the outstretched legs.

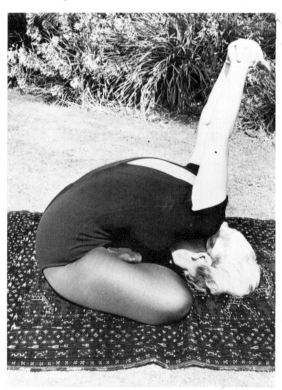

Yoga Mudra—completed.

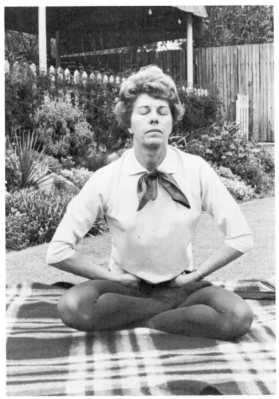

Variation Yoga Mudra—with fists in abdomen prior to bending.

Yoga Mudra

Benefits

The Yoga Mudra stretches the spine and limbers the back and shoulders and removes the tendency to "dowager's hump". It reduces fat on the upper arms and feeds the facial tissues, thus helping to eliminate wrinkles. Last, but not least, it stimulates the bowels.

Method

Sit on the mat in either the Lotus, Half-Lotus or cross-legged position. Put the arms behind the back and clasp the left wrist with the right hand. Inhale, then brace the shoulders and raise the arms up backwards as far as is possible, then exhale and whilst exhaling bend the trunk forward towards the floor and endeavour to place the forehead onto the floor. Maintain the posture for a few seconds with the breath out, then inhale and return to starting position, lowering the arms slowly.

Repeat the exercise, remembering to breathe out as you go down, and to breathe in as you come up.

When you first perform the exercise repeat it three times, then slowly increase the number of repetitions up to ten.

Remarks

It is important to bend forward from the hips and not from the waist. Do not jerk the arms, but press them upwards slowly. The Lotus is the best seat to use for doing this posture as the heels press into the pelvic area and create pressure on the bowels. If you are unable to sit in the Lotus, you may also perform the exercise by placing the fists in either side of the pelvic area and whilst bending forward the fists will have the same effect as the heels. This exercise relieves constipation.

Back Stretching posture

Benefits

This is another exercise which strengthens the spine and keeps it elastic. The Back Stretching Posture is particularly good for the lumbar region of the back and will help to keep you free from lumbago! It also stretches the ham strings of the legs, strengthens abdominal muscles, tones up internal organs and bowels and will help women suffering from constipation.

Method

Lie down on your back on the mat with the arms at the sides. Inhale to sit up, then exhale and slowly stretch forward with the trunk and arms and clasp the insteps with the fingers. Endeavour to drop the elbows alongside the knees and keep the legs straight. Maintain the position for a few seconds, then inhale to sit up, exhale and roll slowly back to starting position. Take a deep Yogic Breath, and then repeat the exercise. The exercise may be repeated up to six times.

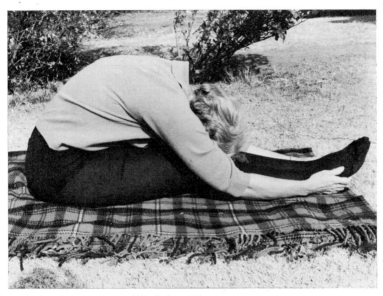

Back Stretching posture.

Remarks

Do not jerk the body, the movements must be slow and deliberate. If it is not possible to take the insteps, then bend forward only as far as is comfortable, trying to improve the posture with practice. When rolling back to starting position keep the movement under control and endeavour to roll on to each vertebra as you slowly lower the back to the floor.

Leg Raising posture

Benefits

This exercise strengthens and flattens the abdomen, thus it is a "must" for those women who have excess fat on the abdomen or muscles which need toning up.

Method

Lie down on the back on the mat and have the hands at the sides, palms down, and feet together. Breathe in and raise both legs simultaneously under control to the vertical position, maintain

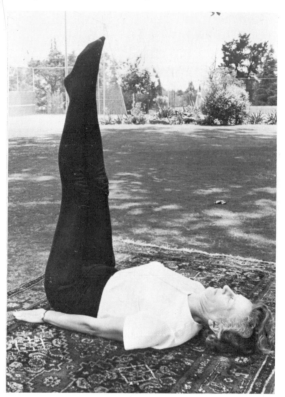

Leg Raising posture.

this position for a few moments, then breathe out whilst slowly lowering the legs to the floor. Take in a deep Yogic Breath and then repeat the exercise. You may repeat the exercise as often as is comfortable.

Remarks
If you experience difficulty in raising both legs simultaneously, then you may practise the posture by raising and lowering one leg at a time.

Beware
This exercise is fairly strenuous and should not be done whilst menstruating, nor should it be done by anyone with a weak heart.

Leg Raising posture with toe holding

Benefits
This is another in the series of exercises which tone the abdominal muscles and organs. All fat tummies, please note! The muscles of the thighs are firmed, middle-aged spread disappears.

Method
Lie down on the back on the mat, hands at the sides, palms down and feet together. Inhale and raise the right leg and the right arm simultaneously, then grasp the toes with the fingers, hold the position for a few moments, then release the toes, exhale and lower the arm and leg simultaneously to starting position.

Repeat the exercise with the left leg, and then finally raise both legs and both arms at the same time.

Remember to take a deep Yogic Breath between repetitions of the complete exercise, and you may repeat the exercise as often as is comfortable.

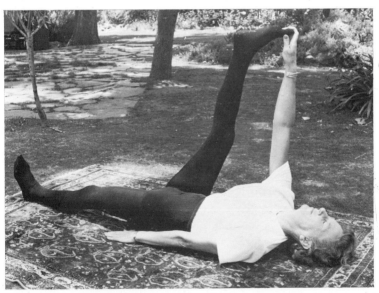

Leg Raising posture with toe holding—first part.

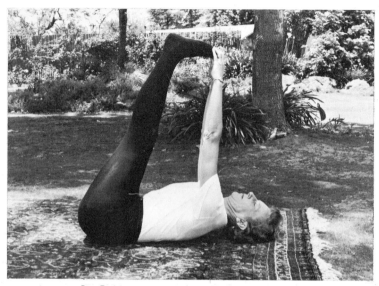

Leg Raising posture with toe holding—completed.

Remarks

Whilst raising each leg individually endeavour to keep the back flat on the floor, as also the remaining leg. When both legs are raised endeavour to keep the buttocks flat on the floor. At all times, keep legs straight. Once again ensure that the movements are executed slowly and deliberately.

Beware

Do not do this exercise whilst menstruating, nor should it be done by anyone with a weak heart.

Scissors

Benefits

This and the next exercise, (the Circles), are for you if you are aiming to achieve a flat and svelte look. They are two of the best possible exercises for the abdominal muscles and will dispose of excess fat as well as strengthen the wall of the abdomen.

Method

Lie on your back on the mat with the hands at the sides, palms

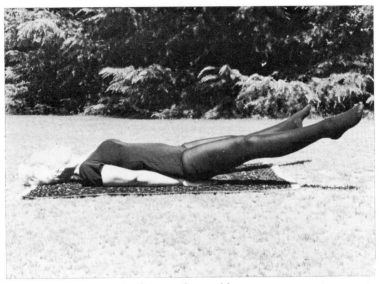

Scissors—first position.

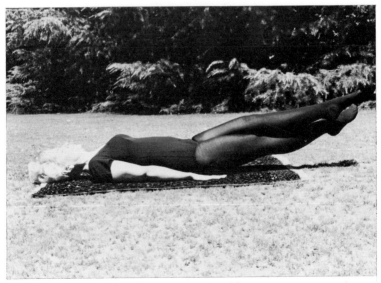

Scissors—second position.

down and feet together. Inhale and half fill the lungs, then raise both legs six inches from the floor, hold the breath and perform the scissors action with the legs for as long as comfortable. Exhale, and slowly lower the legs. Take a deep Yogic Breath and then repeat the exercise. Gradually increase the number of times you repeat the exercise, but do not strain.

Remarks
The nearer to the floor you are able to keep your legs, the more beneficial the exercise. Do not do this, or any of the other abdominal exercises, during menstruation.

Circles

Benefits
This is the other exercise which is so good for the muscles of the abdomen.

Method
Lie on your back on the mat, have the hands at the sides palms down, and keep the feet together. Inhale, then exhale and slowly raise the legs, then inhale and slowly bring the legs down separately in an outward circle to within six inches of the floor, then exhale and raise the legs, inhale and bring the legs down in an outward circle, and continue in this same manner for as long as is comfortable. Take a deep Yogic Breath and then repeat the exercise. Gradually increase the number of repetitions.

Remarks
The smaller the circles, the more beneficial the exercise. Do not do the exercise during menstruation. It is essential to keep the abdominal wall firm and strong, particularly as one gets older, because if the wall should become weak the internal organs tend to sag and drop out of place.

Beware
Once again, do not attempt the above two exercises if you have a weak heart.

Siamese posture

Benefits
Slims the waist, strengthens the lungs and increases their capacity, therefore it will assist women suffering from bronchial troubles. Massages the colon and the kidneys.

Method
Sit down on the mat and fold the legs to the left side of the body keeping the knees flat on the floor. Raise the arms above the head and join the palms together, keeping the fingers pointing upwards.

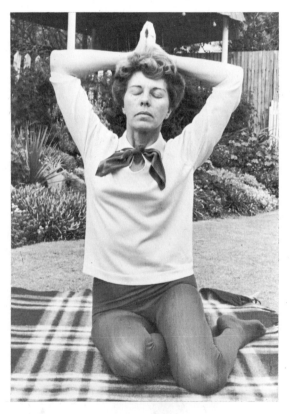

Siamese posture—starting position.

wer the hands and arms and place the hands lightly on top of
head, keeping the hands together and the elbows back.

1. Inhale, then exhale as you bend the trunk to the left towards
   the feet.
2. Inhale as you return to starting position.
3. Exhale and bend towards the feet.

Continue with the exercise for as long as it is comfortable.
Change the legs to the right side and repeat the exercise, bending
towards the right.

Remarks

Do not bend forward. Keep the bend to the side, so that the whole
of the side and trunk is stretched.

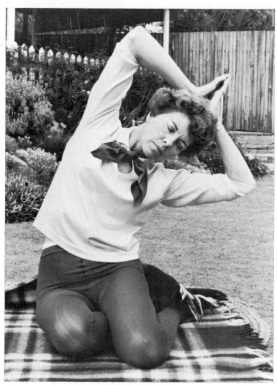

Siamese posture—bending towards feet.

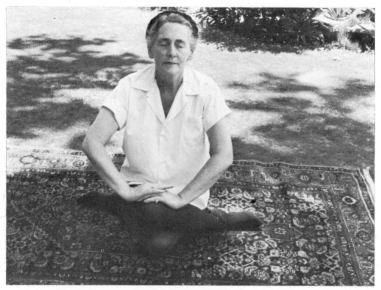

Preliminary to the Cow.

The Cow

Benefits

This is another BEAUTY exercise. It disposes of any "dowager's hump", relieves tension in the back and slims the upper arms. It also stretches the sciatic nerves in the legs and is an excellent exercise for increasing the lung capacity. It benefits the knees, ankles and insteps, and strengthens the trapezius muscles.

Method

Sit down on the mat, legs stretched out. Take the right foot and draw it towards the body and place it underneath the left thigh. Take the left foot and lift it over the right leg and then pull the feet round to the sides of the body. Have the buttocks flat upon the floor, and sit in the triangle formed by the legs.

Now stretch the right arm upwards, reach around the back with the left arm and endeavour to make the fingers of both hands meet behind the back, so that the fingers of the right hand hook over the fingers of the left hand. Inhale and stretch back with the arms, opening up the chest, then tighten the grip of the fingers, relax and breathe out. Repeat this movement three times, then take a deep relaxing breath, release the position, change arms and legs and repeat the exercise with the other leg and arm.

Remarks

As a preliminary to the Cow, you may place the hands with the fingers interlocked upon the crossed legs, then inhale and whilst holding the breath press the knees outwards and down. Relax, change your position and repeat with the other leg uppermost. This exercise increases the effect on the sciatic nerves and stimulates the nervous system.

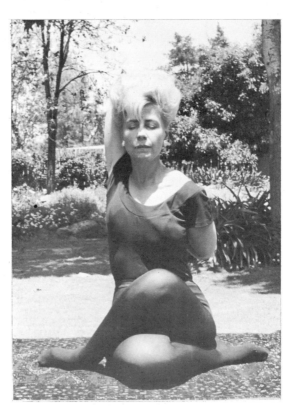

The Cow—front view.

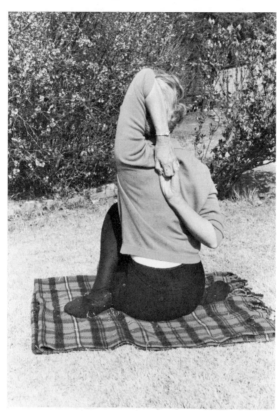

HK. ↳
1 hand
other catch
+ pull.

The Cow—back view.

Beware
Do not sit in either of the positions above for too long if you suffer from varicose veins.

The Camel

Benefits
Some women will find this a difficult exercise to do, but it has such rewarding benefits that it deserves special attention and practice and with perseverance you will be delighted with your

progress. Flabby thighs become firmed, the back and the arms are strengthened, the line of the throat is beautified and all of the inner organs are toned. It will also keep your knees young. It benefits the thyroid.

Method

Sit down on the knees on the mat. Lean backwards and place the hands flat on the floor, fingers pointing towards the knees. Inhale and raise the thighs and abdomen and let the head fall backwards, arching the spine and keeping the arms straight. Hold the position, then exhale and lower yourself slowly to starting position.

When you are able to do the foregoing simpler version of the posture, try to do it by placing the fists of the hands in the soles of the feet and then push the thighs and abdomen upwards, hold the posture and then relax.

Once again you must remember to take a deep Yogic Breath between each repetition of the exercise. The exercise can be repeated up to three times.

When you are able to do the posture with ease try to hold it

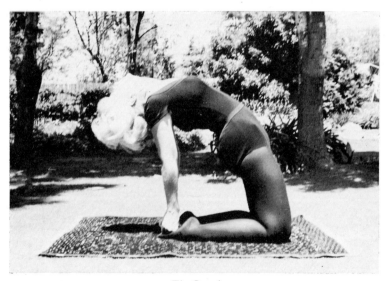

The Camel.

whilst easy breathing and endeavour to increase the time you are able to maintain the final position.

Beware
If you are suffering from an over-active thyroid, do not attempt this exercise.

The Twist

Benefits
This is a very graceful looking exercise and it is one of the most important exercises for the spine, because it gives it an excellent lateral twist. At the same time it tones up the liver and stimulates the adrenal glands. Women who are inclined to be liverish should never omit this exercise from their daily routine, nor should those who suffer from asthma or constipation. It prevents lumbago.

Method
1. *The Starting Position* Sit down on the mat and stretch out

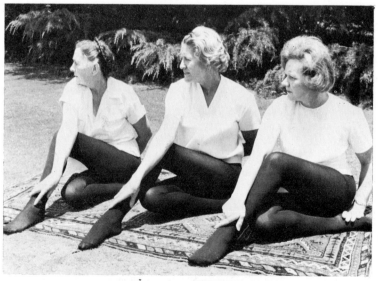

The Twist or Sphinx—first part.
(*The student nearest the camera should have her left hand behind the body, touching the right hip.*)

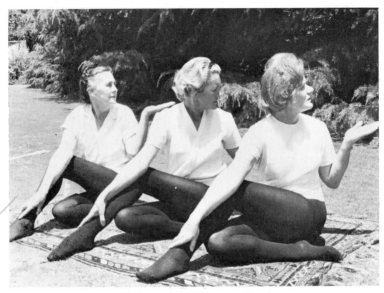

The Twist or Sphinx—completed.

both legs. Draw the right foot up and place it under the left thigh. Lift the left leg and place the foot just in front of the right knee. Take the right arm in front of the left leg and grasp the left ankle with the right hand. Take the left arm around behind the back and rest it lightly on the right hip, whilst you turn the head to the right and look over the right shoulder.

2. The object of the exercise is to twist the whole of the trunk using the arm and knee as a lever, and this you do slowly and carefully by breathing in, breathing out, turning the eyes slightly towards the left and then following with the head. Repeat this movement until you are looking over your left shoulder, then take the left hand from the right hip, tuck the elbow into the side and raise the hand, palm upwards, and point the fingers in the same direction as that in which the eyes are now looking. Use the right arm as a lever against the left leg to really twist the upper part of the trunk as far as is possible to the left.

3. It will not be easy to breathe deeply in this extreme position, so breathe lightly and hold the position for about ten seconds, then slowly unfold and return to the original position by returning the left hand to the right hip, breathing in and out, turning the eyes slightly to the RIGHT this time and following with the head until you are back in the starting position.

Take a deep relaxing breath when you are once again in the Starting Position, then unfold the legs and repeat the exercise by changing over legs and arms and twisting to the opposite side which will be towards the right.

Do the exercise once only on either side.

Remarks

The directions sound more involved than they really are, so it will be a great help if you are able to have someone read the instructions to you whilst you are learning this exercise. As you progress with the Twist, try to hold the posture in its extremity for a greater length of time.

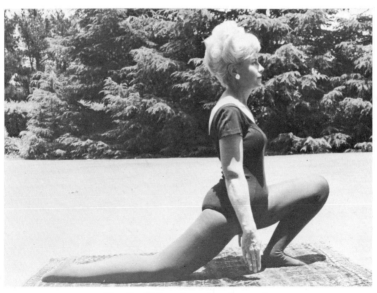

Kneeling Cobra—lowering the trunk.

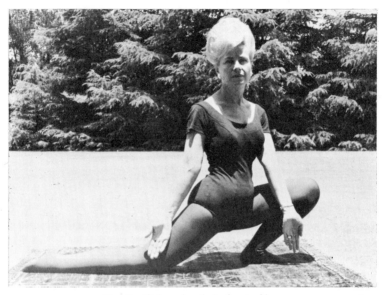

Kneeling Cobra—hands in front of legs.

Kneeling Cobra

Benefits

The adrenals are stimulated, the legs are strengthened and firmed, the backbone receives a lateral twist and the hips are reduced.

Method

1. Kneel down on the mat, then slide the right foot forward and place it firmly on the floor about 24 inches in front of the left knee. Keep the arms close to the body and let the hands hang down loosely.

2. Inhale, then exhale as you lower your trunk down towards the mat whilst transferring the weight from the knee to the foot and trying to touch the floor with the tips of the fingers of each hand. The left leg will be stretched out behind the body, whilst the right foot must be kept FLAT upon the floor and the back must be kept straight.

3. Inhale, return to starting position, then repeat the exercise by exhaling to lower and inhaling to raise, then place the hands

in front of the body, twist the trunk around to the left, exhale
and lower the body. Inhale and return to starting position.
Change legs and repeat the whole of the exercise.

Remarks
Do not lean forward whilst lowering the trunk. The exercise can
be repeated as often as you wish.

The Cobra

Beware
If you are suffering from an over-active thyroid, do not attempt
this exercise.

Benefits
The Cobra will help you to keep your spine young and supple.
The adrenal glands are stimulated and any tensions in the back
will be relaxed. This posture strengthens the muscles of the back,
and it is of great benefit to women's internal organs, thus it will

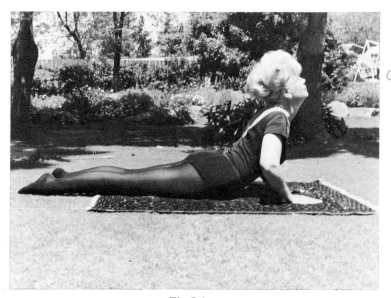

The Cobra.

be of help to women suffering from menopausal or menstrual disorders.

In addition to all of the foregoing benefits, the Cobra will beautify the neck and firm the bust.

Method

Lie down on the abdomen on the mat, chin touching the ground, hands palms down underneath the shoulders. Have the elbows pointing upwards and keep the legs together with the toes pointed.

Inhale and slowly raise the head, shoulders and chest from the floor like a cobra and slowly arch the spine backwards, but keep the lower part of the body flat on the floor so that you will feel the pressure in the small of the back. Maintain this position for a few seconds, then exhale slowly and lower the body until you return to starting position.

Take a deep Yogic Breath and then repeat the exercise. The Cobra may be repeated up to six times, but do not tire or strain yourself.

Remarks

Always perform the movements slowly whilst endeavouring at the same time to raise the trunk as far as you can. DO NOT STRAIN.

The Locust

Benefits

The Locust is a natural follow-on to the Cobra, as whilst the Cobra strengthens the upper portion of the spine the Locust strengthens the lumbar region. The Locust also has a beneficial effect on women's internal organs, thus it should be done by women suffering from menopausal and menstrual disorders. In addition to the foregoing, the thighs and buttocks become firmed and reduced and the respiratory organs become strengthened.

Method

Lie on the floor, face downwards, chin on the ground and place the hands palms up underneath the thighs. Inhale and raise the right leg slowly as high as is comfortable, hold the position for a few seconds, then exhale and return the leg slowly to starting position. Repeat the same movement with the left leg.

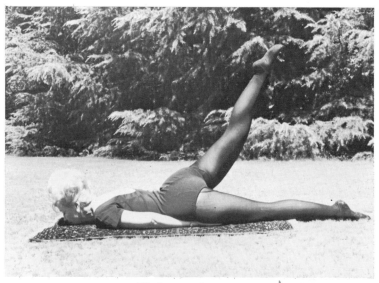

The Locust—first part.

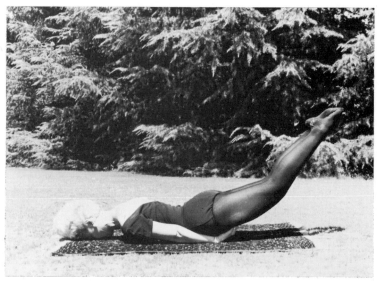

The Locust—second part.

Take a deep relaxing breath and rest for a moment, then inhale and place the forehead on the floor and endeavour to raise both legs upwards and backwards, helping the thighs in their upward movement with the hands. Hold the full position for a few seconds, then exhale and return the legs slowly to the floor.

Rest and take a deep breath before repeating the exercise. The Locust may be repeated up to three times.

Remarks
Do not be discouraged if you find this posture difficult to assume when you first start to practise it. You will strengthen the muscles slowly and will be pleased to see how you improve this exercise.

The Bow
Although this posture is not an easy one to assume, you will experience a great sense of achievement when you have accomplished it.

Benefits
The Bow benefits the entire spine and the sympathetic nervous

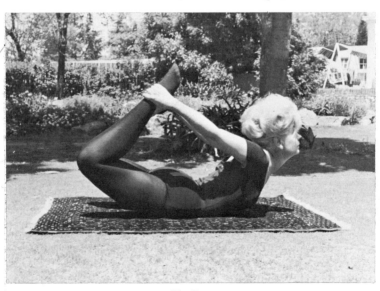

The Bow.

system. It tones up the liver, firms the bust, reduces fat on the abdomen, thighs and hips, and stimulates the bowels. Women suffering from mentrual or menopausal disorders should include this exercise regularly in their daily practice. The Bow is really guaranteed to make you feel on top of the world!

Method
Lie flat on the abdomen, resting the cheek on the mat, and place the hands palms down underneath the shoulders as in the Cobra.

Now inhale and stretch straight up on the arms, then bend your legs at the knees and stretch back with the hands and take the ankles. Pull on your ankles and raise head, trunk and thighs, so that your body assumes a curved "bow-like" posture. Endeavour to hold the final position for a few moments, then exhale and return to starting position, first lowering the knees and feet and then the trunk. Carry out all the movements slowly and deliberately and rest and take an easy breath before repeating the exercise. You may repeat the exercise up to three times, and then as you advance you may prefer to maintain the posture whilst breathing easily rather than repeating it.

Beware
If you have an over-active thyroid, do not attempt this exercise.

The Plough

Benefits
The Plough will give the maximum s—t—r—e—t—c—h to the spine. With age the spine tends to telescope into itself and this will be remedied and prevented with the practice of the Plough. The thyroid gland is stimulated, excess fat on the stomach will disappear, and in general unwanted weight will be reduced. Good also for menstrual and menopausal disorders and for digestive troubles. Regular practice of the Plough will also help to prevent arthritis.

Method
Lie on your back on the mat with the hands palms down at the sides, legs stretched out and feet together. Inhale and slowly

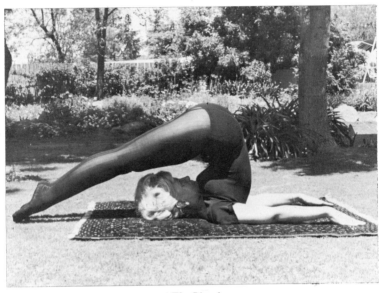

The Plough.

raise the legs to the vertical, then exhale and carefully tip the hips and legs over the head and place the toes on the floor. Keep the legs straight and press the chin well onto the chest. Maintain the position for a few seconds whilst easy breathing. Inhale and lower the buttocks to the floor whilst returning the legs to the vertical position, then exhale and slowly lower the legs to the floor. Take a deep relaxing breath.

Remarks
This exercise may be performed as a static posture (maintaining the posture), or as a dynamic exercise (repeating the exercise). If you choose to maintain the posture, gradually increase the time for holding the final position, and if you wish to repeat the exercise, then increase the number of repetitions from one to six as you progress with your practice.

If, at first, you cannot lower the toes to the floor, take the legs over the head only as far as they will go. At no time must you strain.

The Shoulder Stand

The Shoulder Stand is one of the most wonderful exercises in Yoga, and should never be left out of your daily practice schedule unless you are menstruating.

Benefits

The inverted position of the body in the Shoulder Stand has a profound rejuvenating effect upon the whole system. This position alters the pull of gravitation upon all our organs and consequently is most restful. It enables the heart to rest from the arduous task of pumping all the venous blood back to the heart from the legs

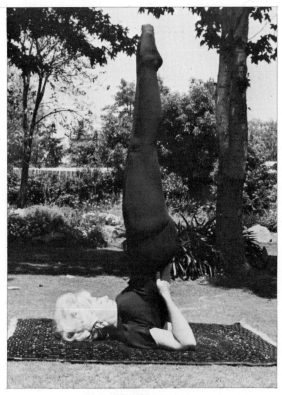

The Shoulder Stand.

and from pumping the arterial blood up to the head. The thyroid and para-thyroid glands are benefited, and consequently all other glands in the body are stimulated. Haemorrhoids and varicose veins will respond favourably to this asana, and it will also strengthen all internal organs and help to prevent prolapse of the uterus. The brain receives a supply of enriched blood and the tissues and muscles of the face are fed, thus reducing the tendency to wrinkles. The Shoulder Stand will also aid in sterility, excess weight, and menopausal and menstrual disorders. Done in the late afternoon when you feel tired, it will rest you and restore your energies.

Method

Lie on the mat on your back, hands at the sides, palms down, feet together. Inhale and raise both legs slowly to the vertical, then exhale and slowly tip the buttocks and legs slightly over and towards the floor whilst bringing the hands to the hips and supporting the body with the hands and upper arms and then stretch the legs and body straight up into the vertical position. It is important that the chin be pressed onto the chest as this creates the necessary pressure on the thyroid. Keep the legs as straight as possible and maintain the posture for as long as comfortable whilst breathing easily. When you are tired and wish to return to starting position, inhale and lower the buttocks to the floor and the hands to the sides, then exhale and slowly lower the legs to the floor.

Remarks

You will derive greater benefits from the posture if you are able to maintain it for a while, rather than by repeating it. For that reason, endeavour to increase your holding time by 30 seconds per week until you are able to hold the Shoulder Stand for five minutes comfortably.

The Reverse posture

This posture is very similar to the Shoulder Stand, except that where in the Shoulder Stand you will endeavour to raise the legs and body to the vertical and to keep them as straight as possible, in the Reverse Posture you keep the legs at an angle.

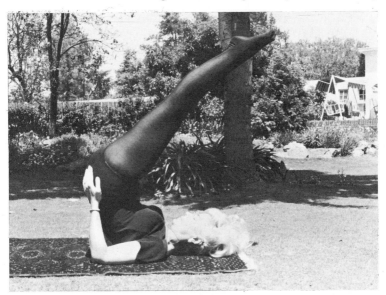

The Reverse posture.

Benefits

The benefits are much the same as the Shoulder Stand, except that there is not quite the same pressure on the thyroid gland. As the Reverse Posture is easier to do than the Shoulder Stand, elderly women and those with stiff backbones are advised to perfect the Reverse Posture before attempting to do the Shoulder Stand. The Posture will help to prevent wrinkles, will restore vitality and will assist in menstrual troubles.

Method

Lie on your back, hands at the sides, palms down, feet together. Inhale and raise the legs to the vertical. Tip the buttocks and legs slightly over towards the head and support the hips with the hands and upper arms and exhale. Maintain this position for a few seconds or for as long as it is comfortable whilst breathing easily. When you desire to return to starting position, inhale and return the hands to the sides and lower the buttocks to the floor, then exhale and return the legs slowly to starting position.

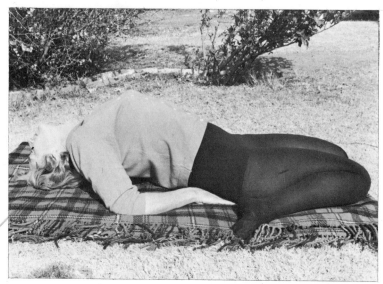

Supine posture.

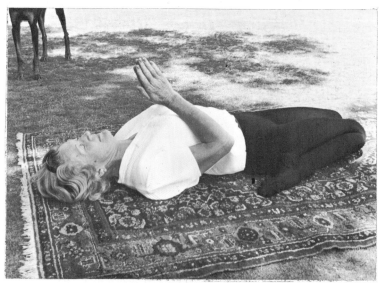

Supine posture—variation.

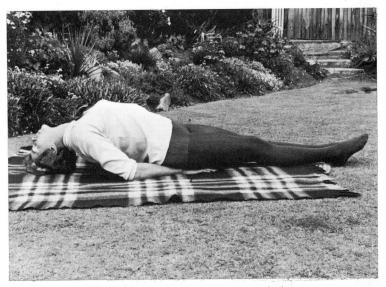

Supine posture—with legs outstretched.

Supine posture

Benefits

This posture should follow the Shoulder Stand and the Reverse Posture, as it relieves any tension across the back and eases the throat. It will enrich the voice, expand the rib cage and lungs, improve the line of the throat, strengthen the small of the back and keep the legs supple. This is a most effective exercise for reducing the excess fat on the thighs. Benefits the glandular system, also the stomach and intestines.

Method

Sit down on the mat between the knees. Inhale and slowly lower the body backwards—first on to the left elbow, then on to the right elbow, then keeping the back arched, lower the top of the head to the floor. Exhale and maintain the posture for a few seconds, or for as long as comfortable whilst breathing easily. When it is desired to return to the sitting position, inhale and push yourself up with the aid of one elbow and then with the other elbow and return to starting position.

This posture is one which should be maintained rather than repeated, so endeavour to build up the time that you hold the posture.

Remarks
If it is not possible for you to sit between the knees, then lie down flat on your back on the mat and place the hands palms down underneath the thighs. Slip forward on to the forearms and arch the back and place the top of the head on the mat, stretching the neck. Maintain the posture for as long as comfortable, then relax and lower yourself to starting position. Doing the exercise this way will not reduce the thighs, but the rib cage and lungs will still expand and the neck and shoulders will still be benefited.

Tranquil posture

Benefits
This is a relaxing and rejuvenating posture. Those women who suffer from insomnia will find the Tranquil posture to be of help if done before retiring.

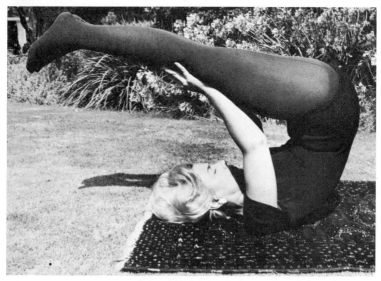

Tranquil posture.

Method

Lie down on the mat, hands at the sides of the body, palms down. Inhale and slowly raise the legs to the vertical, exhale, tilt the buttocks and legs towards the head, raise the hands and support the knees and legs with the arms and hands. Maintain the position and breathe naturally. When the position has been held for as long as comfortable, inhale, lower the buttocks and the hands, and then exhale and slowly return the legs to starting position.

Remarks

It is better to maintain the posture for a period, rather than to repeat it.

The Headstand

I have left the Headstand until last, because I feel that the body should be toned, the muscles must be made responsive and the balance of the body improved by doing other exercises before the Headstand is attempted. To endeavour to do a Headstand immediately you start the practice of Yoga is incorrect. Very few women are used to their heads being below their knees with the consequent flow of blood to the brain and increase in blood pressure, (even when lying down most people use pillows), so endeavour to get the body into a more supple condition and the head and brain used to an inverted position before you attempt to do the Headstand.

If you are unable to do the Headstand for any reason whatsoever, there is no necessity for you to feel that you are not doing Yoga. The Shoulder Stand and The Tortoise will bring you most of the benefits of the Headstand.

Benefits

The Headstand is considered to be the King of Asanas. It brings the blood to the brain, strengthens the arteries of the head, alters the pull of gravitation on the body, rests the heart, strengthens the mind, improves the memory, the powers of concentration, and the condition of the ears and eyes. It will help those women who suffer from migrain, headaches, varicose veins, uterine disorders, asthma, nervousness, insomnia and poor circulation. It will improve the growth and condition of the hair and stimulate and balance the endocrine glands.

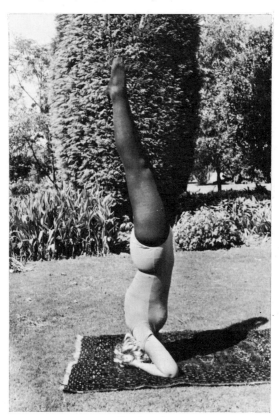

Headstand.

Method

1. Kneel down on the practice mat and make a triangle with the arms on the mat. Interlock the fingers of the hands, keeping the thumbs up and resting the hands on the ridges formed by the little fingers, so that the hands will form a cup in which the head will be supported.

2. Place the frontal portion of the head down on the mat, cup the hands around the head and have the arms and interlocked fingers resting firmly upon the mat.

3. Straighten the knees, keep the toes upon the mat, and walk in towards the head very slowly until the knees are close to

the body and you begin to feel the body balancing on the head.

4. With a slight hop draw up the knees and feet, so that you are balancing on the head and arms, keeping the knees tucked into the body. Retain your balance in this position.

This first half of the exercise must be perfected before you attempt to extend the legs and straighten them into the completed posture.

5. When you have mastered the first half of the exercise and can remain in the half-position with ease, endeavour to straighten out the legs vertically. Do this very slowly and hold the full Headstand for a short while.

6. *To return to starting position*
Return the legs very slowly to the half-position, then gently lower the feet and knees to the floor. Keep the head down on your hands for a short while before sitting back on your heels.

Remarks
Hold the position as long as is comfortable, usually about ten seconds when you first attempt the headstand, and increase the holding time to suit yourself, but do not go beyond ten minutes.

When making your first attempt have someone nearby to assist you to maintain your balance whilst perpendicular, or if that is not possible, attempt the Headstand in a corner so that you will not overbalance and hurt yourself.

Beware
NEVER do the Headstand if you suffer from high or low blood pressure, sinus, catarrh, broken veins in the cheeks, or blood shot eyes caused by weak eye capillaries. Nor should it be done by those with disorders of the thyroid or with heart trouble. Do not take a hot bath immediately before or immediately after the Headstand.

Concluding Remarks

There are many other exercises or asanas and many more variations, (according to legend there are 84,000!) but those given in the foregoing pages are practical, cover all the parts of the body, and are eminently suitable for housewives and career women. You should derive much pleasure and satisfaction in their performance.

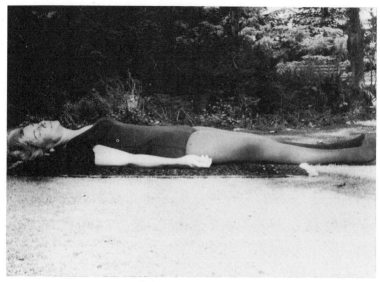

Relaxation—palms up.

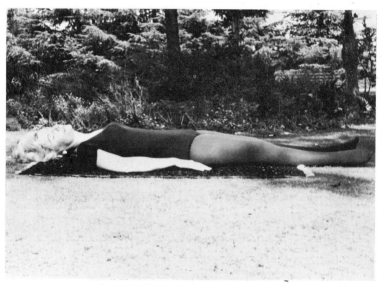

Relaxation—palms down.

Once again I would stress, do the exercises with caution, avoiding all strain and discomfort, and, of course, avoid those exercises which are not suitable for you. Begin with the simple exercises, and MAKE HASTE SLOWLY.

Here is a suggested daily routine for you:

> Limbering
> *Breathing*
> Alternate Nostril Breath
> Deep Yogic Breath
> One of the other Breathing Exercises
> *Exercises*
> A Neck or Shoulder Exercise
> A Spine Exercise
> An Abdominal Exercise
> A Back Strengthening Exercise
> The Stretches
> An Inverted Posture

Vary your exercises and include any exercises which you wish to do to improve any particular condition relative to yourself. In this connection make use of the particulars given under "At a Glance" at the back of the book. Remember to take a short rest between each exercise, and if possible, finish off the exercises with Relaxation, unless you wish to relax at a later time during the day. To learn to R-E-L-A-X is the next important step in your training, so on to Part Two please.

PART TWO

1

The art of relaxation, or how to add years to your life

THE CALL for relaxation today is far more urgent than it ever was. Everyone should know how to relax and all can learn, but it takes practice and concentration. Usually, when women are particularly in need of relaxation they invariably say, "Yes, that's all very well, but I haven't the time." In those last few words lies the cue. "I haven't the time." That is exactly when they MUST MAKE the time. If they fail to do so they are likely to become tense and irritable, and then not only will they suffer but their entire families will also become involved. Who will take care of the family when mother has to go to a nursing home to recover from a nervous breakdown? Realise the importance and value of relaxation and devote at least fifteen minutes per day to developing an art which you will enjoy and which will refresh and restore you and release all nervous tensions.

You may relax indoors or out, and if you cannot possibly lie down you can relax sitting up in a comfortable chair, providing your back and arms are supported and you have your feet flat on the floor. It is naturally more pleasant to relax whilst lying down, and if you have a quiet garden it is delightful to relax in the open air. If this is not practicable, or if there is the possibility of interruption, then relax in your bedroom.

Method
1. Ensure that you will not be disturbed, that the children are taken care of and that if the telephone rings someone will be available to answer it and take messages.
2. Shut your bedroom door, remove your dress and shoes and any tight clothing, put on a light gown and then lie down flat on your back on a rug on the floor. Be sure there is no draught

blowing from underneath your door and cover yourself with
a light blanket. If you have a hollow back it will help to place
a small cushion under the knees.

3.   Do not be tempted to practise your relaxation on the bed—
lying on a soft bed will cause the muscles to become tense, it
is far more beneficial to relax on a hard surface like the floor.
You will relax yourself in bed before going to sleep at night,
but your daily practice must be done on the floor.

When you first learn how to relax, it is advantageous to tense
all the muscles of the body, as this seems to help beginners to let
go during actual relaxation. So, make yourself quite comfortable
on the floor and then:

(i) take in a deep breath, clench the muscles of the toes,
breathe out and let go,

(ii) take in a deep breath, tense the muscles of the legs, breathe
out and let go,

(iii) take in a deep breath, tense the muscles of the buttocks,
breathe out and let go.

Continue in this manner, tensing in turn the shoulders, fingers,
arms, jaws and muscles of the face.

After you have learned the art of relaxation, you will be able to
leave out these preliminaries.

NOW, prepare to really relax and LET GO, and to indulge
and enjoy yourself for the next fifteen minutes.

Deep Relaxation

Remain where you are on the floor, have the hands at the sides,
palms down and the elbows slightly crooked so that the weight of
the arms and hands is taken by the floor. (You may, if you prefer
it, lie with the hands palms up, but I prefer the former method.)
Let your feet fall outwards and let the small of your back drop
down towards the mat. Let your head roll until you find a comfortable position without strain. Close your eyes, drop the lower
jaw so that the teeth are parted, and rest the tongue lightly against
the inside of the bottom teeth. This helps to relax the jaw and
throat. Shut out all distracting sounds and try to still the mind.
Concentrate solely upon relaxing the body, do not make any
movement because if you do you will break the sequence of the

relaxation—you must lie perfectly still. Deep Relaxation is commenced with deep breathing, but after this initial breathing let the breath take care of itself so that when you are fully relaxed the breath will be almost non-existent.

Draw in a full, deep, Yogic Breath, drawing in the Prana or life force through the toes, up the legs, up the body, through the arms right up to the head, and then exhale, letting the breath sweep right down to the toes again, carrying with it all tiredness, tensions and worries. LET GO as you breathe out. If it helps you, you can picture this breath as a wave gently washing up over you as you breathe in, and then sweeping down back over you and carrying away with it all tensions as you breathe out.

Repeat this deep breathing routine three times, and then after the last exhalation, begin to relax the body. Start by trying to relax the toes, and then work slowly right up the body. Repeat to yourself, slowly and silently:

"TOES . . . . . RELAX . . . . . TOES . . . . . RELAX", then proceed to the heels,

"HEELS . . . . . RELAX . . . . . HEELS . . . . . RELAX", then proceed to the ankles,

"ANKLES . . . . . RELAX . . . . . ANKLES . . . . . RELAX", then let the FEET go, feel them HEAVY and RELAXED.

Carry on in this way by going to the calves, then to the knees, then to the thighs, then let the legs go, HEAVY AND RELAXED. . . . Then go to the buttocks, the Solar Plexus, the chest, the shoulders, the back, then let the body go, HEAVY AND RELAXED. . . . Proceed to the fingers, the hands, the wrists and the arms. Let them go, HEAVY AND RELAXED. . . . Next go to the throat, let the lower jaw drop, relax the muscles of the face, letting the cheeks sag and the eyelids droop, smooth out the lines of the face and keeping the eyes closed relax them and let them slip backwards into the head turning the gaze to the spot between the eyebrows, keep the eyelids quite still and closed. Let the whole head go and finally relax the back of the neck where all tensions gather. Let the whole body sag from the crown of the head to the tips of the toes. BE HEAVY AND RELAXED. . . . Feel the body sinking into the floor, and the floor pressing upwards. Try to still the mind, letting all thoughts run down. Withdraw all the nervous tensions from the body and feel it become weightless, as light as air. Finally, shut yourself off completely, turn within and find the peace and tranquillity which lies within you. (Remember, you are the mistress of your soul—only you can find your inner harmony, and only you can shut out irritations and peace destroying emotions.)

Lie quietly in this way for as long as you wish, and then when you are ready to return to activity, take in a deep Yogic Breath, once again drawing the Prana or life force through the toes, right up the legs, through the body, through the arms, right up to the head, but this time as you exhale concentrate on and direct all the life-giving energies to the Solar Plexus. The Solar Plexus as you have previously learned is the seat of our nervous energies, and it is here that we wish to store the Prana which we are drawing in. Repeat the deep Yogic Breath three times, and then S-T-R-E-T-C-H. First stretch with the arms right up above the head and down with the heels, then roll over onto the side and stretch, then roll over to the other side and stretch.

Finally, lie on your back and rest for 30 seconds and then sit up slowly. You will now feel completely restored and ready to take on life again.

Whilst relaxing, if you wish, you can visualise some particular thing of beauty—a favourite flower, a colour, or picture the waves lapping the sea shore and then receding. As your ability to relax improves, you will feel so delightfully light and weightless that you will be unable to tell where your limbs are resting. You will experience the delightful sensation of floating and perhaps you will drift off to sleep. Sleep whilst relaxing is the most refreshing sleep of all. You will awaken quite suddenly—your eyes will just open and you will be wide awake once more but feeling completely refreshed and not heavy as one usually does from a sleep during the day. When you become expert at relaxation, you can decide in advance how long you wish to relax and you will not need any outside assistance to waken at the expiration of the time. For example, if you lie down at 3.15 p.m. and wish to relax for 30 minutes, then exactly on the dot of 3.45 p.m. your eyes will open automatically and your relaxation will end. This will happen quite naturally and without any effort on your part. However, when you first start to practise relaxation, you can arrange to be called at the expiration of the desired time, or you can set a small alarm clock in the room, but do not keep taking a peek at your wrist watch. That is no way in which to relax!

If you are working during the day, then relax when you return home. Be quite definite about it and allow nothing to distract you. Set this time apart for yourself, even if you have a great deal to do when you return home. It will only mean that things will be attended to 20 minutes later, but more important, it will also mean that you will feel 100 per cent fitter and more like doing what you have to do. It will also mean dividends in health for you—instead of feeling tired out and exhausted, you will feel refreshed and ready to enjoy the company of your family.

2

Health Practices

DO YOU wake up in the morning, stretch out an arm for your early morning tea or coffee and drink it and pretend that the world and the day doesn't exist? Sorry, but this is an offence against better health and bodies. Yoga insists on cleanliness of the body, both inside and out, and for this reason, nothing, but absolutely nothing must be taken into the system before the teeth and tongue have been cleaned!

Mouth
During the night various waste deposits are formed on the tongue, and if these are swallowed again they cause a toxic state to develop in the body. So it is of the utmost importance when you waken in the morning that you get out of bed and proceed straight to the bathroom. Clean your teeth thoroughly, brushing them up and down and not across, and then proceed to clean your tongue. This is done by scraping the tongue with a teaspoon and then thoroughly rinsing out the mouth. Then, and only then, may you proceed to enjoy your early morning cup of tea. Ideally, you should begin the day with a glass of lemon juice and tepid water, unsweetened, but if you cannot take the lemon juice without any sweetening, then add a teaspoon of honey. The lemon juice alkalises the system and helps the bowels to perform their task efficiently.

Nose
Next, it is necessary to clean out the nose properly. To do this the easy way, purchase a small nasal douche from the chemist. It looks rather like a small elongated glass duck and costs very

little. Fill the nasal douche with lukewarm water to which a little salt and bicarbonate of soda have been added, then insert the "beak" portion into one nostril whilst holding a finger on the inlet on the top of the douche. When the beak is securely in the nostril, lift the finger from the inlet and the lukewarm water will slowly filter into the nostril and down the back of the throat. When it reaches the back of the throat remove the nasal douche, bend the head forward and allow the water to come into the mouth, so that it can be ejected into the washbasin. Repeat with the other nostril and as often as desired.

You will be amazed to see how much dust has collected at the back of the nostrils, where no amount of blowing will remove it. This practice also strengthens the membranes at the back of the nose and helps to prevent colds. If you do have a head cold, this system of cleaning the nose will help to clear up the cold. Finally, gently massage the root of the nose.

Ears

Naturally you will always wash the ears gently every day, but also make it a habit to massage behind them daily too. This will loosen the wax and it will work its way upwards so that it can be removed easily. Please do not stick all sorts of odd things into the ears. Hairpins are intended for the hair, not for the ears. If wax is visible, remove it by using the little cotton wool sticks that are intended for ear cleaning and are sold by chemists, or use the little miniature scoop which is now being marketed for the same purpose.

Eyes

Our eyes are very sadly neglected and badly treated. They are on duty constantly, but receive very little reward or regard. Make it part of your morning toilet to bathe the eyes regularly with a weak solution of salt and tepid water. This will strengthen them and keep them bright and clear. During the day you should rest them periodically by blinking and also by "Palming". An explanation of how to do "Palming" is given with the series of Eye Exercises in Part One, and the exercises themselves should also be done whenever you have a few minutes to spare.

It is a very sound idea whilst you are relaxing to rest the eyes as well by placing over the closed lids pads of cotton wool which have been dampened with witch hazel, or place a slice of cucumber over each eye.

Beauty and health are very closely related, particularly when it comes to the eyes, so be sure that you have adequate rest and exercise combined with a sound diet, and, of course, no eyes will ever be truly beautiful unless the soul within is beautiful too!

To obviate wrinkles forming round the eyes always use a heavy eye cream regularly at night, but be very careful that you do not pull the sensitive skin around the eyes whilst applying the cream. Pat it on very gently with the ring finger. Always wear a hat whilst in the bright sun and do check with your occulist if you have eye strain or headaches.

Inner Cleanliness
Inner cleanliness is vital. In exactly the same way as one's exterior deserves attention, so does one's interior. Yoga lays specific stress on this part of cleanliness. For this reason, various rules of diet are laid down, and in the East certain postures are performed for cleaning the intestines. When you consider that the alimentary tract is approximately 27 feet long from mouth to rectum, and that the colon itself, which is the part of the system where the waste matters of the body collect before being discharged in the normal way, is approximately 5 feet long, you will more readily understand why it is so necessary to keep the tract in a clean and healthy state. If waste matters are allowed to remain in the colon either through constipation or laziness, the toxic by-products are absorbed through the intestinal walls into the bloodstream and general toxemia results. This will mean a poor appetite and digestion, a muddy and spotty complexion, dull eyes, halitosis and a general lack of vitality. As you wash the skin to remove all dirt and grime, so you should flush out the colon with water in order to keep it clean. In the average adult person there are many old and hardened remnants in the various little kinks in the colon which have formed over the years, and they will remain there unless they are flushed away. This clogged condition will be a constant source of poisons entering into the bloodstream, so do not be afraid to take an occasional enema. It is assumed that you

are familiar with the equipment needed for an enema and how it is taken, but if you are in any doubt consult your physician. Use tepid water and first clear out the lower bowel by taking a pint of water and then take four pints for the full enema. If you suffer from chronic constipation it is more sensible to take an enema than to persistently strain at a motion.

Constipation

This is one of the major ills of modern civilization. Pick up any newspaper or magazine and in it you will find advertisements for various patent cures for constipation. As people get older their digestive systems slow down, and if they lead sedentary lives and eat incorrectly the position becomes greatly aggravated. If you do suffer from constipation Yoga will help you to overcome it if you will perform the exercises regularly and if you follow the Yoga way of eating. The exercises which will do the most for you in helping you to establish regular bowel movements and to keep the alimentary tract toned are the STOMACH LIFT, the BACK STRETCHING POSTURE, the YOGA MUDRA, the SQUAT-TING POSTURE, the COBRA, the LOCUST, the SWAN and the SIDEWAYS SWAYING POSTURE. Most women find that the bowels will move about an hour after performing exercises selected from the foregoing.

Here too, are some additional ways in which you can help your system to revert to normal:

1. Always respond at once to the call of nature—do not put off your visit to the toilet to a later time.
2. Drink plenty of water between meals (not iced water).
3. Endeavour to train the bowels to move at a regular time each day, preferably in the morning, and in order to help them to do this, take an enema once a week at the same time in an effort to establish regularity of movement. Once the bowels are moving satisfactorily you can leave out the weekly enema and only take it occasionally.
4. DO NOT TAKE PURGATIVES
5. Eat plenty of fruit and vegetables, taking as much as possible in the raw state. Eat cherries, currants, figs, grapes, mangoes, pawpaw, peaches, prunes, strawberries, asparagus, beans,

cabbage, cauliflower, maize, cucumbers, lettuce, green peas, radishes, spinach and tomatoes. (Not all at once, of course!)

6. Eat wholewheat bread as this will act as roughage.

7. Drink milk—it helps to maintain the health of the colon.

8. Boil onions and drink the liquid in which they were boiled. This will act as a laxative. If you do the same with cabbage it will also have the same effect.

9. Soak prunes overnight and then take them together with the liquid before breakfast.

10. Watch the quality and quantity of food eaten. Do not overeat. If you do have an occasional lapse then make sure that the following day you eat as little as possible, concentrating on fruits, salads, juices and water.

The Bath

The skin is more than just an outer covering to the body. Its condition reflects the state of health of the body, and it acts as a respiratory organ and assists the kidneys in their work of throwing off waste materials. Consequently a daily bath is a must, but do ensure that the water is not too hot. Have a pleasantly warm bath and then run in a quantity of cold water before you have finished bathing in order to tone up the skin. During the dry winter months it is advantageous to put a little bath oil into the water to keep the skin from drying out. Use a rough towel to dry yourself, and then rub yourself down vigorously with the hands and finally slap yourself with the palms of the hands. When slapping the legs allow the muscles of the calves and thighs to relax. Use a moisturising lotion in the dry months of the year and pay particular attention to the hands, arms, legs and feet. Finally, as a little touch of feminine luxury, spray the body lightly with cologne—this is most refreshing in summer.

Vaginal Douche

Internal feminine hygiene is good common sense, but make the douche of plain warm water or warm water and a little salt. Do not use disinfectants.

Sun and Air Baths

It is most beneficial to remove the clothes and take an occasional air or sun bath. If you live in a sunny climate you will almost certainly spend some time in a bathing costume in summer and so absorb the health giving rays of the sun. However, great care should be taken to ensure that the skin is not overexposed with the resultant sun burn. Be moderate in your sun bathing. Some skins are very sensitive indeed and over-exposure can be dangerous. Do remember to wear a hat when out in the sun, as too much sun dries out the natural oils in the skin and can cause premature wrinkles. Wear sun glasses to protect the eyes.

If you are unable to take the sun out-of-doors, it is a good practice to expose the whole body to the light and air occasionally and this can be done in the privacy of your own bedroom, particularly if it is a warm room. Do not allow yourself to become chilled.

Bear in mind that the sun's rays at the middle of the day are not so beneficial as those in the early morning or the late afternoon.

Hair

Most women today are conscious of their hair and know it to be women's crowning glory. A good "hair-do" will do wonders for morale as well as for looks. However, for hair to look really fabulous it must be shining, alive and healthy. Hairdressers cannot do much with poor material.

The condition of your body will be reflected in your hair—poor, run down body, will mean poor, miserable looking hair. A healthy, vital, body will reflect in lustrous, lovely hair. So take care of your hair by keeping the body toned through your Yoga exercises and breathing, keeping the system clear and eating the right foods. Eat plenty of green and yellow vegetables, fruit, dairy products, fish and meat, (especially liver and kidneys), wheatgerm and yogurt.

The postures which bring the blood to the head, thus helping the scalp and hair to remain healthy, are the Chest and Arm Stretch, the Jack Knife, the Tortoise, the Yoga Mudra, and the Shoulder Stand and its variations.

Keep your comb and bristle brush scrupulously clean and finally, choose a good hairdresser who will look after your hair. If you prefer to set your own hair, have it cut professionally, wash it regularly once a week with a good shampoo, rinse well and dry in the sun if possible.

Be sure to include onions in your diet—they help the hair to grow!

3

Beauty comes from within—or,
what to eat

THERE were two women engaged in earnest conversation and self-inspection as can only be done in the intimate atmosphere of the hairdressing salon. Number one said, running her fingers through her rather lifeless looking hair, "I wish it would grow! And look how thin it's becoming!" "Well," said her friend, "I have the same trouble. Probably old age! Let's have something to eat, it's nearly lunch time." An apprentice was called over and despatched to the nearby café, and five minutes later the two ladies were busily munching white bread rolls, whilst balancing a sweet cold drink and a doughnut on their knees.

Old age indeed! Here was the reason for their lifeless hair and sallow looks. YOU ARE WHAT YOU EAT. Think before eating, ask yourself, "What is this going to do for me? Is it going to nourish and revitalise my system, or is it going to clog it up, make my complexion sallow and spotty, my eyes and my hair dull and lifeless?" Be as exacting about what you eat as you are about choosing a new dress. You are not a human vacuum cleaner! Select from the aristocrats of foods. See that you have plenty of fresh vegetables, (raw and cooked), fruit, eggs, milk, cheese, yogurt, nuts and honey. Do not eat white bread and white sugar, but eat delicious wholewheat bread and brown sugar. Do not eat other foods made from white flour, (cakes, pastries, macaroni, spaghetti, noodles, etc.), polished rice, tinned foods, fried food, over-spiced food and made-over food. Take fruit juices, milk or yogurt in preference to sweet cold drinks. In so far as meat is concerned, Yogis are strictly vegetarians, but it is not necessary for us who live in the West living normal lives as housewives and mothers to follow this rule. Should you wish to become a vegetarian, do so. After an initial period whilst the body adjusts itself to a meatless diet you will find that you will feel much better than you did when you were a meat eater. However, this is a matter for you to decide personally. Good wholesome food, simply prepared, is healthy food. Steamed vegetables are far more nutritious than overcooked vegetables smothered in sauces and creams. Do not fry foods and try not to use too many spices, salt, flavourings, fats, sugars, etc. Do not eat foods which have been cooked and constantly reheated, neither should you eat foods ice cold or excessively hot. Try to take a certain quantity of raw vegetables and fresh fruit every day, and do not eat at all hours of the day throughout the day. Most women will be happy with two meals a day, that is breakfast and dinner, but if this is not suitable, then eat three LIGHT meals a day. Don't eat unless you are hungry, and sometimes give your whole system a rest through fasting.

It is better not to take alcoholic beverages. This is not only for health reasons but also for figure reasons. There are no advantages to be gained from taking alcohol. It causes a toxic condition of the body, blood and brain, and puts on unwanted poundage. Don't take too much or over-strong tea, and, of course, you are better off if you are able to leave out coffee.

Recognise yourself in any of the DON'TS above? Then determine to alter your pattern of eating! Add years to your life and renewed vitality to your system by changing to the health giving and revitalising foods. It will take a little time for you to accustom yourself to your new way of eating, but you will begin to feel so much more alive that you will wonder how you ever ate the over-refined and devitalised foods with such misguided gusto.

Concentrate on fresh vegetables and fruit grown in organic soil without chemical fertilizers or poisonous sprays.

You must endeavour to eat a BALANCED diet consisting of a variety of fruits, vegetables, cereals, sugars, fats, milk, eggs, honey, yogurt, meat and fish. If you do not wish to eat meat or fish, then milk, cheese, eggs, wholewheat products, almonds, cabbage, soya beans, spinach and tomatoes taken in adequate quantities will supply the necessary proteins.

For sparkling eyes, a glowing complexion, lovely teeth and nails and prolonged youth and health, eat

Apples	Celery	Marrows	Parsnips
Asparagus	Cucumber	Naartjies	Potatoes
Apricots	Dates	Nuts	Raisins
Bananas	Fresh Figs	Oranges	Radishes
Beetroot	Gooseberries	Peaches	Radishes
Beans (green)	Grapes	Pears	Spinach
Carrots	Grapefruit	Pumpkin	Squash
Cherries	Lemons	Pineapples	Strawberries
Currants	Lichis	Pawpaw	Tomatoes
Cauliflowers	Lettuce	Plums	Turnips
Cabbage	Mangoes	Prunes	Watermelons

In fact, all fruits and vegetables.

For a youthful-looking and slim figure

You may eat all vegetables excepting potatoes, and all fruits except grapes, raisins, mangoes, bananas and dates. Concentrate on apples, cherries, figs, gooseberries, grapefruit, lemons, lichis, naartjies, oranges, pineapples, plums, pawpaw and watermelon.

Foods to avoid are all cereals, (including bread), wheat products, (cakes, biscuits and pastries), and all sugars, (sweets, chocolates, jams, syrups, jellies, ice cream, puddings). Cream, whole milk and butter should also be left out, but you may take buttermilk and skimmed milk.

Specially recommended for teeth, nails, bones and heart are grapes, dates, raisins, asparagus, cabbage, celery, lettuce, spinach, tomatoes, green peas, carrots, parsnips, turnips and potatoes.

WATER should be taken freely at all times between meals. It cleanses the system and should be taken daily at the rate of one glass of water to every stone of body weight. (One stone equals 14 lbs.) The water should not be out of the refrigerator, that is iced, but should be taken at its natural temperature. Water has a taste and is one of nature's delightful gifts to man. We do not drink with meals because by doing so we dilute the gastric juices of the stomach and thus make digestion difficult.

Here is a list of the essential health vitamins, and here too, are some of the foods in which they are found:

Vitamin A   This is the vitamin that prolongs life, is necessary for growth, helps with the development of bone and teeth, helps to prevent disease and colds, supplies energy, makes the eyes sparkle and keeps the skin and hair beautiful. It also enables the glands to function properly, particularly the adrenals and thyroid. It is found in BUTTER, CHEESE, EGGS, CARROTS, GREEN AND YELLOW VEGETABLES and YELLOW FRUIT, MILK, LIVER, KIDNEYS and COD LIVER OIL.

Vitamin B complex   This group prevents tiredness, supplies energy, and is necessary for the health of the nervous system. It promotes growth, helps to improve the appetite and digestion and improves the body's resistance to skin diseases. It keeps the skin, eyes and hair healthy (prevents greying). It is found in LIVER, KIDNEYS, WHEAT GERM, MEAT, POTATOES, EGGS, MILK, PEANUTS, VEGETABLES, FISH, FRUIT, YOGURT and YEAST.

Vitamin C   Vitamin C means strong teeth and bones, resistance to infection, a glowing and healthy skin, healthy mucous membranes and muscular tissues. It will help to keep you youthful, improve your eyes, and the endocrine glands. It is found in LIVER, CITRUS FRUIT, VEGETABLES, GUAVAS, PINE-APPLES, PAWPAWS, CABBAGE, TOMATOES and MILK.

Note! Vitamin C is easily destroyed by heat, therefore it is essential that vegetables are not overcooked. To guard against the loss of Vitamin C whilst cooking green vegetables and to retain the colour, add a little lemon juice to the water.

Vitamin D   Vitamin D is essential for strong bones, gleaming and healthy hair and strong teeth and nails. This really is a Beauty Vitamin! It is found in SUNLIGHT, COD LIVER OIL, EGGS, LIVER, BUTTER, MILK, CREAM and CHEESE.

Vitamin E   This vitamin is believed to influence the reproductive process. It is found in GREEN VEGETABLES, WHOLE CEREALS, VEGETABLE OILS, CARROTS, TOMATOES, NUTS, EGG YOLK.

Fats   These animal and vegetable fats are the source of essential fatty acids necessary for the normal functioning of the body. They are the most concentrated form of heat and energy. Animal fats are found in BUTTER, CREAM, CHEESE and MEAT FAT, whilst vegetable fats are the fats and oils found in VEGETABLES, NUTS, OLIVES and AVOCADOS.

Carbohydrates   Carbohydrates, which include the starches and sugars, provide heat and energy for the body. Starches are found in cereals, (bread, rice, maize, etc.), potatoes and DRIED LEGUMES. Sugars are found in FRUIT, HONEY and SYRUPS.

Rules for happy eating

1. Sit up straight. Do not be in a hurry whilst eating.
2. Chew your foods well and do not eat when you are angry or upset in any way. Food taken in these circumstances will only lead to indigestion.
3. Ensure that you have clean, pleasant surroundings and that your table companions are pleasant.
4. Digestion begins in the mouth and your stomach performs a very important function and has plenty of work to do. Consequently, see that the teeth, tongue and saliva do their share of the work before the job is passed on to the stomach. CHEW YOUR FOOD WELL. You must pay particular attention to starches, as these should be converted to glucose by the saliva in the mouth before they are swallowed. If this is not done they will ferment in the stomach and cause gas.
5. Do not over-eat. Eat to satisfy the stomach and hunger, not the eye and appetite.
6. Eat fresh vegetables and fruit every day. Uncooked fruit and a raw salad should be eaten daily.
7. Endeavour to buy or pick your vegetables so that they are fresh daily. Handling and storage makes them wilt and destroys vitamins.

Recipes

Here are a few recipes for you to try in your new pattern of healthy eating. Ensure that all ingredients used are the best obtainable and as fresh as possible. Use brown sugar, not white, whole-wheat flour and sea or vegetable salt.

Bircher Muesli

This is the famous breakfast dish served in the Bircher Clinic in Zurich, Switzerland. It is a raw fruit porridge and makes a most nutritious dish. Fruit is the main ingredient in the Muesli, and you must not use more oats than is specified in the recipe. The apples must be tart and juicy and must be coarsely grated, and the final dish should be light, not stiff and heavy. Make the Muesli just before eating. The rolled oats or oatmeal must be soaked overnight, but do not soak the quick cooking varieties. It is preferable to use the rolled oats or oatmeal.

Here is the basic recipe:

Ingredients per person
1 LEVEL tablespoon rolled oats, (or 1 level dessertspoon medium oatmeal) soaked for 12 hours in 3 tablespoons water
1 tablespoon lemon juice
1 tablespoon sweetened condensed milk
1 LARGE apple (or 2-3 small ones)
1 tablespoon grated hazelnuts or almonds

Method
1. Mix lemon juice and condensed milk to a smooth cream.
2. Add to oats, stirring well.
3. Wash apples and grate coarsely into mixture, stirring frequently to prevent discolouring.
5. Sprinkle nuts on top of mixture and serve immediately.

Delicious Wholewheat Bread

Ingredients (MAKES TWO 1 LB. LOAVES)

2 lb. wholewheat flour	1 tablespoon sunflower oil
2 heaped tablespoons wheat germ	1 tablespoon molasses
2 level tablespoons powdered skim milk	1 heaped tablespoon salt
2 cakes yeast	1 tablespoon honey
	$1\frac{1}{4}$ pints tepid water

Method

Put one tablespoon sugar in half cup warm water and add the 2 cakes of yeast, mix and allow to stand for 15 minutes.

Grease two 1 lb. bread tins.

Mix dry ingredients together, make a well in the centre and pour in the yeast, add the honey and molasses mixed with half the quantity of tepid water. Blend. Then add the remaining water and the oil and mix. Put into greased tins to rise in warming oven for approximately 1 hour or until it doubles its bulk, then bake at 400°C. for 10 minutes, and 375°C. for 50 minutes.

Date Scones

2 cups wholewheat flour
4 teaspoons (level) baking powder
2 tablespoons brown sugar
1 cup chopped dates

2 tablespoons butter
1 tablespoon wheat germ
1 egg in cup of milk and
    water

Blend dry ingredients, rub in butter and add beaten egg, milk and water mixture. Mix lightly, turn out and flatten slightly and cut out scones with pastry cutter. Bake at 450°C. for 10 to 15 minutes.

Wholewheat Pastry

Half-cup boiling water
1 cup oil

2 cups wholewheat flour
$\frac{3}{4}$ teaspoon salt

Pour boiling water over oil and blend. Sift flour and salt and stir into liquid. Mix well. Chill for half-an-hour, then divide dough into halves and roll on pastry cloth. Makes two 9-inch crusts.

Vegetable Appetiser

3 cups tomato juice
1 stalk celery and leaves
2 sprigs parsley
3 tablespoons brewers yeast

$\frac{1}{2}$ lemon and rind
$\frac{1}{2}$ green pepper
$\frac{1}{2}$ onion

Cut up celery, lemon, green pepper (remove seeds), and onion. Place all ingredients in liquidiser and blend thoroughly.

Crisp Salads

Gather your salad greens and fruit from your garden just before your require them, or, if you have no garden and have to buy them, buy them as fresh as possible. All vegetables and fruit should be washed carefully and then drained. If you do wish to store them, keep them in the refrigerator in plastic bowls with tight fitting lids, or in plastic bags. Try to buy vegetables and fruit grown in naturally composted soil. Avoid all fruit which has been sprayed with insecticide.

Do not prepare the salad ingredients hours before you need them, and prepare the salad as short a while as possible before serving it. Make it your custom to serve a fresh salad at least once per day, and in summer time it is a good idea to serve it as the main course. If you do, then you should add cheese, eggs, meat or fish.

Cabbage Salad

$1\frac{1}{2}$ cups very finely shredded cabbage
1 red and 1 green pepper (optional)
1 small onion, finely sliced
Approx. $\frac{1}{4}$ pint cooked salad dressing
Salt and pepper
Large pinch paprika
3 or 4 tablespoons finely grated cheese

Method

Shred cabbage finely and stand for about half-an-hour in iced water to crisp. Drain well and dry. Slice the peppers very finely and remove the seeds. Combine cheese with salad dressing and dress the salad. Pile in a salad bowl and serve very crisp.

Cooked Salad Dressing

$\frac{1}{2}$ teaspoon salt	1 tablespoon sugar
1 egg	4 tablespoons butter
1 small level teaspoon dry mustard	4 tablespoons lemon juice
	2 tablespoons cream

Method

Melt butter in top of double boiler, add egg lightly beaten along with all other ingredients, except cream. Cook until thickened.

Remove from heat and pour into bowl to cool slightly, add cream. Chill and use as required.

Some Different Salads

Here are a few salad combinations which you might like to try as they are a little different from the usual tomato and lettuce.

When making French Dressing, substitute lemon juice for the usual vinegar or, if you wish, you can use grapefruit juice and lemon juice combined. A touch of crumbled Roquefort cheese also adds to the flavour of the dressing.

1. Serve grated carrot, cauliflowerettes, orange segments and French dressing.
2. Fill avocado pear halves with grapefruit segments and French dressing.
3. Fill avocado pear halves with diced pineapple, apple and celery and French dressing.
4. Fill avocado pear halves with peeled grapes, halved, and French dressing.
5. Stuff tomatoes with shredded pineapple, grated cabbage and French dressing.
6. Stuff tomatoes with grated cucumber, celery, pecan nuts and onion.
7. Serve chopped tomato and avocado pear, chopped onion and lemon juice.
8. Serve fresh sliced peaches with lemon juice, cottage cheese and mint.
9. Serve lettuce, pineapple, orange segments, cream cheese and sour cream and paprika.
10. Serve radishes, cucumber, green pimento (remove seeds), spring onions (all sliced), cream cheese, yogurt, lettuce, sprinkling of black pepper and paprika.
11. Serve sliced hardboiled egg, grated celery, carrot, sliced radishes, cucumber, covered with dressing made of yogurt, little paprika, 1 teaspoon lemon juice, 1 teaspoon orange juice, pepper and one teaspoon finely chopped parsley.

Supper Dish

Take pieces of toast and spread on each a mixture of cottage cheese, salt and pepper and some grated nuts. Grate together apples and carrots and mix a little lemon juice, sugar and very little oil. Spread this mixture on top of the cheese and decorate each piece of toast with a slice of lemon and a cherry.

Baked Carrot and Cheese

$\frac{1}{4}$ cup butter   dash pepper
1 finely chopped onion $\frac{1}{4}$ teaspoon celery salt
$\frac{1}{4}$ cup flour   12 cooked finely chopped carrots
1 teaspoon salt $\frac{1}{2}$ lb. grated cheddar cheese
$\frac{1}{4}$ teaspoon mustard powder   3 cups buttered fresh breadcrumbs
2 cups milk

Method

Melt butter in a pan. Add the onion and cook slowly for 2 minutes. Stir in flour, salt and mustard. Then stir in milk. Cook slowly whilst stirring until the mixture is thick and smooth. Add the pepper and celery salt. Now place a layer of carrots in a casserole, followed by a layer of cheese. Repeat until both ingredients have been used up, ending with a layer of carrots. Pour the sauce over the carrots and sprinkle the crumbs on top. Bake for 20 minutes at 350°C.

Diet during Pregnancy

Continue to eat normally as outlined on the foregoing pages, i.e. fresh fruits, vegetables and salads, eggs, cheese, fish, meat in moderation, wholewheat bread, honey, yogurt, and plenty of milk, preferably two pints per day.

Avoid all fatty, fried and spiced foods, all white flour products, white sugar, cakes, puddings, biscuits and all sweets, chcolates and sugary cold drinks. Do not take any alcohol. Drink plenty of plain water.

To sum up

Combine good food, good eating habits, your Yoga exercises, breathing and relaxation, and you must strike the Health and Beauty Jackpot!

4

Fasting for pleasure

DO NOT OVEREAT! This is one of the greatest trans-gressions in an affluent society. Everyone has a built-in appetite control, and when this signals "ENOUGH!" you should stop eating at once, no matter how tempting the foods remaining on your plate appear. Remember the reference to vacuum cleaners —YOU want to maintain your health and youthful looking figure.

Periodically it is a good idea to give your entire digestive system a rest through fasting, but this suggestion is not always welcomed by women. Habits die hard and most exclaim, "But that is not good for you! You must eat!" Here it must be pointed out that if you are suffering from a duodenal ulcer, or if you are very much underweight, then you would be quite right, but most normally healthy women will benefit from a fast lasting from one to three days.

Why should you fast?
The blood stream is purified, the organs of digestion are rested, the brain becomes more alert and all the senses of smell, sight and taste improve. Nature herself demonstrates that sometimes it is better not to eat. Have you not noticed that when animals and young children are feeling off-colour they will not eat again until they are well? Fasting is a natural means of eliminating poisons and wastes from the body and will leave you feeling completely rejuvenated.

To fast means to go without food or liquids with the exception of water. Most women can manage to do this for one day, but find it difficult to continue beyond that stage on water only. To help you to prolong the fast you may take lemon juice with the water, or, if you prefer it, orange juice.

How to fast

Naturally, it is not a good idea to undertake a fast when you have several dinner engagements to fulfil, or when you are going to have a lot of exhausting work to do. Choose a time when you will really be able to devote your attention to yourself, and when you will not have husband and family fussing around mother because for some unknown reason she has become quite demented and is refusing to eat! Perhaps you will be able to organise it when your husband goes off on a business trip and the children are otherwise occupied. Make up your mind for how many days you wish to fast, and then spend your fasting days doing the things you want to do. Now is the time to make the new dress from the pattern you have been treasuring, or to experiment with paints and canvas, or to give yourself a good home facial, and on the last day go and have a new hair-do. Make sure too, that you give full time to your daily relaxation. This inner and outer treatment should make you feel and look completely rejuvenated.

One-Day Beauty Fast

If you have put on unwanted weight, are uncomfortable in your clothes and feel that your silhouette is not quite what it should be and that your system is sluggish, then go on a One-Day Beauty Fast regularly once a week, until you have succeeded in putting matters right. Excess weight is not becoming, neither is it healthy. The heart has an increased burden placed upon it, whilst your feet and legs will also suffer. The ankles will swell if you are carrying a great deal of excess weight, and very often varicose veins form.

The One-Day Beauty Fast consists of taking one 8-oz. glass of fresh orange juice as often as you wish throughout the day. At least six glasses of water should also be taken, but nothing else whatsoever.

It is also a good idea to follow this Beauty Fast whenever you have over-indulged in a lot of extra rich food.

Other Diets

If for some reason you do not wish to leave out all food and take water or juice only, then you may go onto a "FRUIT DIET", or a "MILK DIET", or a "FRUIT AND MILK DIET". These diets will also cleanse and revitalise the system, and may be followed from one to three days.

The Fruit Diet
Drink plenty of water and eat apples or pineapple for breakfast, lunch and dinner. The water, of course, will be taken between meals.

The Milk Diet
Take one 8-oz. glass of orange juice upon arising, and then take as much milk as you wish throughout the day.

The Fruit and Milk Diet
Take one 8-oz. glass of orange juice upon arising, then for breakfast eat apples and drink one 8-oz. glass of milk.

Lunch: Oranges and pawpaw and one 8-oz. glass of milk.

Dinner: Oranges and pawpaw and one 8-oz. glass of milk.

You may also take a glass of milk mid-morning and mid-afternoon.

If you have a weight problem you can substitute skimmed milk for the whole-milk mentioned in the above two diets.

Breaking the Fast
To break the fast or diet, (if it has lasted for more than one day), reintroduce other foods gradually. Make your first meal an apple, skin and all, and ensure that you chew it well. Then for the following three meals you could take a thick vegetable soup, and after that revert to your normal diet in small quantities.

You will find that you will be more particular about your diet after a fast. You won't want to dive into forbidden sweets and pastries, because you will feel so healthy and full of energy that you will want to continue feeling that way. Consequently, it is often a good idea if you want to lose weight and yet cannot discipline yourself to leave out the fattening foods to go on a short fast first, and then afterwards you will find it no problem to eat the right foods and to leave out the wrong ones!

5

How to ensure a peaceful night's sleep

I T IS surprising how many women suffer from insomnia and how many resort to taking sleeping pills in order to get to sleep. Yet sleep should come naturally to everyone at the end of a day's activities, as naturally as night follows day. Now, why is it that difficulty should be encountered in following one of nature's simple and restorative processes? In most cases of insomnia when the head is put on to the pillow instead of sweet release coming from sleep the activity of the mind seems to become accelerated. The would-be sleeper begins to toss and turn trying to find release, but instead of a slowing down and a gentle lulling, every worry and half-worry crowds into the mind and begins to jostle for preferential treatment. With peculiar clarity these worries now appear to become gigantic and insoluble and far worse than when viewed in the light of day.

How has this situation come about? Usually through nervous tension which, in turn, has been caused by allowing worries to assume impossible proportions and in the end they get completely out of hand. Nervous tension works hand in glove with worry, so nervous tension increases worry. Worry reciprocates and increases nervous tension, thus we have the never ending vicious circle and the position slowly but surely degenerates and eventually a bottle of sleeping tablets becomes indispensable.

Why do people worry? Worry can and does cause depression and disease. It causes asthma, migraine, ulcers and heart trouble, so why do we worry? Life in the 20th Century is full of difficulties, so if you are faced with, or are in what appears to be an impossible situation fraught with problems on all sides, there is more sense and reason in trying to find a solution rationally than by letting your emotions take control, creating tensions, and tearing you into small pieces.

One of the first things you must do is to learn to RELAX. We all know the old maxim of taking a breath and counting up to ten. There is a lot of sense in this. Instead of getting worked up to fever pitch about something, take a deep breath in and let go and refuse to become upset. Instead, sit down and determine to think about the matter or situation sensibly. First of all, establish just what all the implications of the position are, and then decide whether the problem is really that important; then take a view on whether the drastic end result visualised will ever come about. Once you have satisfied yourself as to its importance and the probability of its happening, then decide what to do about it, and when you have done this, be business-like and proceed along those lines and then dismiss the matter from your mind.

That is the only practical way for dealing with problems—there is no point in continually "worrying" your problems. Sort them out, decide what to do, and then leave them alone. Remember it is impossible to go through life without having any difficulties to overcome—fire hardens and moulds the metal!

If you don't learn to become rational and practical about your worries, you will develop into a worrier. You will have a perpetual worried feeling and worried expression and you will find yourself treating everything, even pleasure, as though it were some insurmountable difficulty.

Once you have freed yourself from that worried feeling and have accepted life for what it is and have learned to approach your problems rationally, you will find that you are no longer subject to nervous tension. Without nervous tension, when you put your head down onto your pillow you will fall asleep naturally and you will sleep peacefully.

Here are some other suggestions which will help to ensure that you have a restful and not a sleepless night:

1. See that your bed is comfortable, with a level, firm, mattress.
2. Have bed covers which are light, warm, and sufficiently large so that they do not slip off you during the night.
3. Ensure that your night clothes are comfortable. Do not wear anything tight.

4. See that the room is darkened properly with no irritating lights shining through the windows or the door.

5. Ensure that you have proper ventilation and sufficient fresh air. This means that you should have a window open at all times, even in cold weather.

6. Have your bed running from North to South in line with the magnetic currents of the earth. Sleep with your head to the North if possible.

7. If a bath soothes you, take a pleasantly warm bath before retiring. (Some women find a bath at night makes them restless. If so, take yours in the morning.)

8. Do not go to bed immediately after a heavy meal. If you suffer from insomnia it is preferable to have your main meal in the middle of the day, and then have something light to eat in the evening.

9. Do not have a loudly ticking or chiming clock in your bedroom.

10. Take care to see that you go to bed in a relaxed frame of mind. Do not go to bed angry or distressed. Endeavour to rectify matters before retiring.

11. Finally, when you get into bed, let yourself sink down comfortably and then relax. Work through the whole body, beginning with the toes and ending with the head and mind. Let your mind dwell on something pleasant, and before you realise what has happened, it will be morning!

It is not the quantity of sleep, but the quality of sleep which matters. Some people can sleep all night and wake up in the morning feeling completely exhausted. Their sub-conscious minds remain alert and active throughout the night. This is because they cannot relax. Try and train the mind and body to relax and to let go completely. When you get into bed discard your thoughts with your clothes.

Many people do not require as much sleep as others, and as you advance in years you will probably find that you also do not require as much sleep as you did when you were younger. Get to know your own sleep requirements.

The Yoga postures will help you to release tensions, and as you progress with Yoga you will become more relaxed in your body and mind and attitude to life. Problems and difficulties which seemed impossible to overcome will assume their correct size.

The postures particularly recommended for relieving tensions are the Head and Neck Exercises, Shoulder Rotation, Rolling Ball, Chest and Arm Stretch, the Tranquil Pose, Shoulder Stand, and most important of all DO NOT FORGET DEEP BREATH-ING AND RELAXATION.

6

Yoga and age

YOGA can and does help to keep you youthful! Normally, as women advance in years, their bones begin to stiffen and their muscles become rigid. Skins, through lack of proper circulation, lose their peach bloom and lines appear. Energies flag and various "isms" and "ituses" appear. Yoga is the perfect answer to age. The postures are designed to keep the body youthful, irrespective of age. As you will have learned by now, the internal organs are toned and massaged, the circulation is stimulated, the nerves are soothed, the brain and skin are fed with oxygen-rich blood, and above all, the endocrine glands are kept in tip-top order. All this adds up to glowing health!

This may still sound too good to be true, but all this can be achieved, providing of course that you are persistent in your practice. You will not achieve anything if you practise Yoga for six weeks and then forget all about it! You must make Yoga part of your life. It has even been known for grey hairs to disappear and not with the aid of the hairdresser, either!

The endocrine glands or ductless glands have a profound effect upon the youthfulness, health and appearance of the body, as well as upon the state of mind and attitude to life. If the glands fail to work efficiently, the balance of the body is thrown out and the ageing process sets in. Therefore, you will realise how essential it is to keep them in good working order by ensuring that they receive an adequate supply of rich red blood and energy through deep breathing and exercise combined with the resultant improved circulation and body tone.

These glands are often referred to as "ductless" because they release the hormones which they secrete directly into the bloodstream. Each gland has its own set of functions to perform, but at the same time they are closely inter-related and if one gland is not functioning efficiently, it can throw the whole system out of balance, and this can mean illness, depression and changes in weight. For example, if the thyroid is over-active, it results in nervousness, tension, loss of weight and an overstimulated pulse rate, whilst an under-active thyroid causes fatness, apathy, depression and sluggishness.

The names of the glands are:

> The Pituitary—situated in the head
> The Pineal—also situated in the head
> The Thyroid—situated at the base of the throat
> The Para-Thyroids—situated below the thyroid
> The Thymus—situated high in the chest
> The Adrenals—situated just above the kidneys, and
> The Sex Glands, (the Ovaries in women)—situated in
>   the abdominal cavity.

Between them the glands control our rate of growth, weight, the flow of the blood-stream, our personality, mental capacity, sexual development, energies, enthusiasms, nervous temperament and appearance.

Here is a list of Yoga postures you should do regularly in order to keep the Endocrine System healthy and functioning properly:

Gland	*Posture*
Pituitary and Pineal	The Tortoise
	The Supine Posture
	The Shoulder Stand
	The Reverse Posture
	The Headstand
Thyroid and Para-thyroids	The Shoulder Stand
	The Reverse Posture
	The Supine Posture
	The Plough
	The Bow
	The Camel
	The Headstand
Adrenals	The Cobra
	The Locust

The Bow
The Twist
The Supine Posture
The Ovaries   The Shoulder Stand
The Reverse Posture
The Cat Hump
The Special Series for Women
The Stomach Lift
The Camel
The Eagle

Menopause

During menopause certain glandular disturbances take place in the body. Some women pass through this period of life with ease, whilst others become subject to irritability, depression and nervousness. Should you fall into the latter category, recognise the symptoms for what they are and make up your mind to adopt a calm and philosophical attitude; everyone goes through the same readjustment. The menopause is discussed and written about far more freely today than it was years ago, consequently women understand what is taking place and realise that although there are changes in the body, they are still women, wives and mothers. Throughout nature everything passes through different phases— there is the spring, the summer, the autumn and the winter, and so it is with life. Everything and everyone changes too with the passing of time, but there is also beauty and fulfilment.

With the menopause, the glandular disturbance seems most commonly to result in heavy depression, so as an antidote try to develop new interests or a hobby. Try oil painting if you have never done it before, learn a new language, endeavour to grow your own vegetables if you have the space in your garden. Perhaps your own depression could be submerged by helping someone less fortunate than yourself. Endeavour to meet people and to keep your mind stimulated. Now, more than ever before, is the time to pay great attention to immaculate grooming and to your personal appearance. Practising the Yoga postures, the deep breathing and the relaxation will help to ease the tensions, and eating well balanced meals with plenty of raw salads, wholewheat bread, fruits and vegetables assist the body over this trying time.

The Shoulder Stand, the Reverse Posture, the Cobra, the Plough, the Locust, the Supine Posture and the Special Series for Women will be of particular benefit to you.

You may also derive mental peace from reading various uplifting works. Here is a piece which I recently came across in an American magazine. It is taken from a work called *Desiderata* by an American poet of the 1920's named Max Ehrmann.

> Go placidly amid the noise and the haste, and remember what peace there may be in silence. As far as possible without surrender, be on good terms with all persons. Speak your truth quietly and clearly; and listen to others, even the dull and ignorant; they too have their story.
>
> Avoid loud and aggressive persons; they are vexations to the spirit. If you compare yourself with others, you may become vain and bitter; for always there will be greater and lesser persons than yourself. . . .
>
> Be yourself. Especially do not feign affection. Neither be cynical about love; for in the face of all aridity and disenchantment, it is as perennial as the grass. . . . Nuture strength of spirit to shield you in sudden misfortune. But do not distress yourself with imaginings. . . .
>
> Beyond a wholesome discipline, be gentle with yourself. You are a child of the universe no less than the trees and the stars; you have a right to be here. And whether or not it is clear to you, no doubt the universe is unfolding as it should. Therefore be at peace with God, whatever you conceive Him to be. . . . With all its shams, drudgery and broken dreams, it is still a beautiful world. Be careful. Strive to be happy.

Here is another small piece from the Sanskrit *The Salutation to the Dawn*

> Look to this day,
> For it is the very life of life.
> In its brief course lie all the verities and realities of your
>   existence:
> The glory of action,
> The bliss of growth,

The splendour of beauty,
For yesterday is but a dream and tomorrow is only a vision;
But today well lived makes every yesterday a dream of
  happiness, and every tomorrow a vision of hope.
Look well, therefore, to this day.

Menstrual Disorders

Many menstrual discomforts will respond to the regular practice
of Yoga, and in particular the following postures will prove helpful:
The Shoulder Stand, the Cobra, the Bow, the Plough, the Locust,
the Eagle, the Stomach Lift and the Special Series for Women.
Relaxation and deep breathing are invaluable for reducing tension.
As mentioned previously, it is not advisable to do any of the
abdominal exercises whilst menstruating nor should any of the
inverted postures be done. At this time concentrate on the
breathing exercises, the simpler head, arm and leg exercises, and
most of all, on relaxation.

Feet

Unconsciously, our faces reflect the condition of our feet. Indeed,
aching feet can cause wrinkles! Consequently, wear the correct
size shoes—never, never wear shoes that are too small for you—
see that the arches have proper support and that the heel fits
snugly. Do not wear extra high heels regularly. Wear shoes with
sensible heels during the day and keep your high heels for "glamour"
occasions. If your work necessitates a lot of standing, try not to
remain rooted in one spot for too long at a time. Endeavour to
keep the feet moving, as in this way you assist the circulation of
the blood and will help to prevent swollen ankles.

If your feet are aching at the end of the day from the heat, too
much standing or pounding of city pavements, bathe them in hot
and then in cold water alternately for about ten minutes. Then do
the Shoulder Stand and you should feel completely refreshed.
Remember to do the Ankle Rotation and Foot Stretch, and the
Toe Balance to strengthen the feet.

Thinking Young

Keep your mind active and alert, and do not allow yourself to get into the habit of thinking "old". Open your mind to new ideas and new methods—in fact this is far more important as you grow older than when one is younger. How often do we hear, "But don't be so old-fashioned, mum!" The world and its generations change constantly, so it is useless trying to make everything and everyone conform to what you used to do when you were young. Try to be understanding—understand why people do the things they do and try to see their point of view. Rejoice with them in their pleasures and successes and be genuinely sympathetic with their heartaches and sorrows. Avoid irritability and develop a calm and tranquil mind. If you allow yourself to become irritable it sets up a chain reaction and what started out as your own lack of control ends up in a great deal of unhappiness and unpleasantness for all of your contacts and members of your family.

Take all that life has to offer and enjoy it, but at the same time restore the balance by putting something back into it. If you radiate good thoughts, words and deeds, you will find that people reciprocate automatically, and so a beneficial and pleasant chain of reactions is started. There are people of course who seem to derive pleasure in being ill-tempered and bad mannered. If it is your misfortune to come across this type during your daily activities, be pleasant and refuse to allow yourself to be distressed by them. Remember that you are the controller of your emotions—only what you allow to penetrate can influence you.

As we read in *The Salutation to the Dawn*, we should try to live each day to the best of our ability. In this direction it is foolish and wasteful to wait for next week, or next month, or next year, or when the children are older. Time passes all too quickly, and before you realise it the autumn and even winter of life will be here. The spring and summer will have gone, and with them the many irreplaceable joys that those ages bring. The children will have gone, there will be an empty swing in the garden, the cupboards will contain forgotten dolls and toy trains. So make the most of everything whilst you may, then when winter comes you will have the glow of memories of a full life to keep you warm, and instead of living a life of regrets you will go on to savour the delights which the autumn and winter have to offer.

Personal appearance has a profound effect on your mental outlook. Give time and attention to your hair, complexion, hands, clothes and shoes. Keep the body as daintily fresh as your underwear. Choose your clothes carefully and with interest, and avoid all tight clothing, particularly tight foundation garments. It is far better to improve the figure through exercise and correct diet than it is to squeeze any odd bulges you may have into tight corsets!

During the hot months of the year it is essential to have the air circulating freely around the body, so wear light, loose clothing. In the colder months it is also better to have light, warm clothing rather than heavy thick layers of garments.

There is no need to become a slave to fashion, but do not go to the other extreme and never try anything new. Wear a new colour occasionally and although you may be quite convinced that you know what style suits you, there is no reason why you should not try something different. Keeping to a rigid form in anything means that the mind has remained rigid and inflexible, and everyone knows how ageing that is! It is more advisable to buy one dress with good basic cut and style, than it is to purchase three badly cut ones made of poor material. They will soon become out of shape and shoddy looking.

Hands are supposed to be the "give-away" to age, but they need not be. Cream them regularly at night and manicure them at least once per week. If you are a keen gardener, never forget to wear gardening gloves, and if you have any particularly rough work to do use a barrier cream, or once again, wear gloves. Also learn to use your hands gracefully and avoid "old" making mannerisms. Vital energy should be conserved and not expended on fidgety and unnecessary gestures.

Keep your skin youthful and glowing by taking good care of it. You must eat the right foods, and that means plenty of fresh green and yellow vegetables, fruits, salads, dairy products, organ meats, fish, wheatgerm and yeast, and bear in mind that iron rich blood will mean a peaches and cream complexion, so include greens like spinach, parsley, watercress and cucumbers in your diet. Most women in the Mediterranean countries have good skins and I think this is due to the oil which is in their diet, so try to take a little sunflower, peanut or olive oil daily.

The next important step in the care of the skin is to cleanse it well. Cleanse it thoroughly and regularly every evening before going to bed by using a reliable cleansing cream on the face and throat. If you prefer to use soap and water, ensure that the water is not too hot or too cold, and that the soap is very mild. Never leave stale make-up on the face.

After cleansing the skin, you must nourish it by using a recommended skin food and applying it lightly to your face and neck. If you wish you can make a good skin food yourself by mixing together 1 oz. sweet almond oil together with one tube of lanolin. Mix this well and use it as required.

Apply make-up lightly, so that it looks as natural as possible. Never use a heavy make-up because it can be very ageing, particularly excess rouge or eye make-up. Even the faces of little girls can appear years older when they are made up for a fancy dress party! Experiment with a change in make-up from time to time as fashions change in make-up as they do in dress, but do not go to extremes.

Smokers will have to take extra care of the skin, because heavy smoking usually causes the skin to assume a greyish tinge and it becomes wrinkled and lined more quickly than in the cases of women who do not smoke. It is even more important than ever that you have sufficient exercise to stimulate the circulation and get the blood to the tissues of the face. Daily exercises, breathing and walks are a must for you. You must be most fastidious about cleansing and nourishing the skin, and you should take an occasional face pack and an occasional face steaming.

Slices of fresh tomatoes applied to the cheeks whilst resting will stimulate the blood and give you rosy cheeks! Here is a face pack that will impart a youthful glow to the skin. It is made by dissolving one teaspoon of sugar in a little rose water, and then adding that mixture to one tablespoon of honey. Spread on the face, relax and then wash off after ten minutes by using tepid water and then splashing with cold. If the face pack appears to be too liquid, you can add a little Fuller's earth.

If you live in a hot and dry country, always wear a hat or use a sunshade whilst out in the sun.

We have discussed the care of the hair under "Health Practices" but do remember to change your hair style occasionally. Nothing looks more "old hat" than a hair-do which has become perennial because someone once said years ago that it did something for your eyes or profile! Eyes and profiles alter, so should hairstyles!

Sit, stand and walk gracefully. Carry yourself tall with your head up, your back straight, your rib cage high and your hips tucked under. Be assured that as the years pass you will continue to enjoy life to the full, and that, in fact, Yoga will prove to be YOUR KEY TO THE JOY OF LIVING.

At a glance

Abdomen   Scissors, Circles, Stomach Lift, Bow, Raised Leg
   Postures, Trunk Backward Bend, Stretches
Arms   Chest and Arm Stretch, Camel, Wide Angle Posture Sitting
Arthritis   Plough
Asthma and Bronchial Complaints   Anti-asthma exercise,
   Locust, Fish, Headstand, Shoulder Stand, Twist, Siamese
   postures, (standing and sitting)
Back   All the Back Strengthening Exercises, Cobra, Fish, Twist,
   Rolling Ball, Bow, Locust, Kneeling Cobra, Wide Angle
   Stretch Sitting
Balance and Concentration   Eagle, Stork, Toe Balance
Bust Line   Bust Line Improver, Cobra, Bow, Camel
Constipation   Mudra, Back Stretching Postures, Locust, Cobra,
   Stomach Lift, Shoulder Stand, Squatting Posture, Bow,
   Twist, Sideways Slip
Endocrine Glands   Bow, Cobra, Camel, Reverse Posture,
   Tortoise, Supine Posture, Shoulder Stand, Stomach Lift,
   Special Series for Women, Eagle, Locust, Twist, Cat Hump,
   Headstand
Figure   All of the exercises and all of the breathing exercises
Hair   Jack Knife, Tortoise, Shoulder Stand, Chest and Arm
   Stretch, Headstand
Hips   Sideslip, Kneeling Cobra
Insomnia   Relaxation, Rolling Ball, Yogic Breathing, Headstand
Legs, Feet, Toes, to strengthen   Ankle Rotation and Foot
   Stretch, Limbering, Toe Balance, Cow, Fish, Wide Angle
   Standing and Sitting, Stork, Tortoise, Rabbit, Supine,
   Locust

Liver and Kidneys Twist, Swan, Bow, Sideways Slip, Rabbit, Kneeling Cobra, Siamese Postures

Lumbago Twist, Locust, Back Stretching Postures and Back Strengthening Postures

Menstrual and Menopause Disorders Relaxation, Locust, Bow, Plough, Shoulder Stand, Reverse Posture, Cobra, Semi-Cobra, Back Stretching Posture, Fish, Stomach Lift, Eagle, Series for Women, Cat Hump, Headstand

Pregnancy Half-Lotus and Lotus, Series for Women, Cat Hump, Squatting, Dynamic Back Strengthener, The Bridge, Relaxation Breathing

Post Natal Shoulder Stand, Scissors, Circles, Cobra, Swan, Relaxation and gradually introduce all the other exercises

Relaxation and Tensions Rolling Ball, Neck and Shoulder Exercises, Relaxation, Tranquillising Breath, Yogic Breathing

Spine Rolling Ball, Bow, Cobra, Semi-Cobra, all the Back Stretching and Back Strengthening Exercises

Uterus and Ovaries Plough, Eagle, Cobra, Special Series for Women, Cat Hump, Bridge, Cow, Shoulder Stand, Reverse, Trunk Backward Bend

Varicose Veins and Haemorrhoids Shoulder Stand and all the inverted postures

Sciatica Jack Knife, Wide Angle Posture Sitting, Cow

Waistline Siamese Postures, Stretches, Twist

Wrinkles Anti-wrinkle, Chest and Arm Stretch, Jack Knife, Mudra, Shoulder Stand, Tranquil Posture, Reverse, Tortoise

Index to Breathing Practices and Exercises